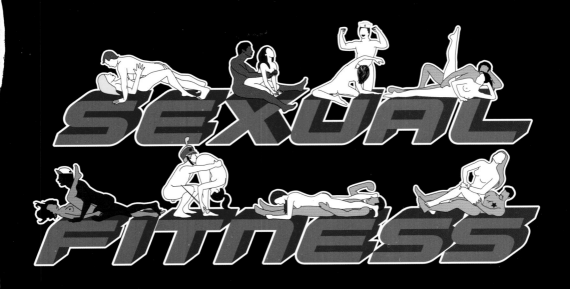

SEXUAL FITNESS

THE ULTIMATE GUIDE TO PUMP WHILE YOU HUMP, TONE WHILE YOU BONE AND SHRED IN THE BED

D.J. Gugenheim, Marc Fellner-Erez, Anat Erez-Fellner and Lee Asher

REMEMBER THE "GOOD" OLD DAYS?

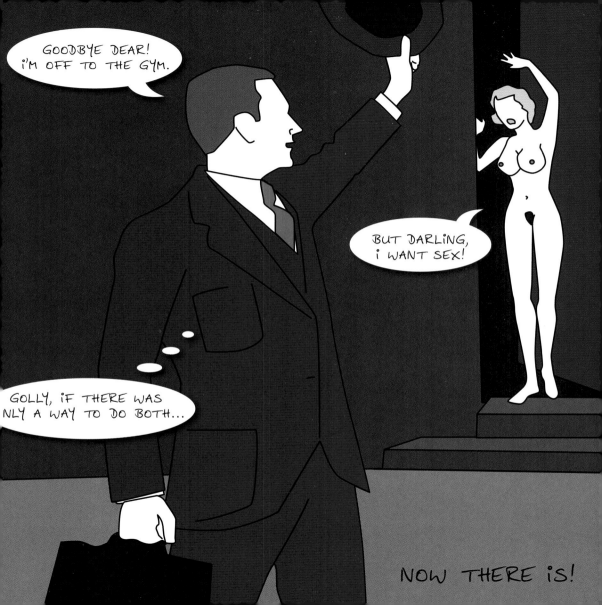

www.stmartins.com
www.sexualfitness.co

Library of Congress Cataloging-in-Publication Data Available Upon Request

ISBN 978-1-250-04114-2 (paper over board)
ISBN 978-1-4668-3729-4   (e-book)

St. Martin's Griffin books may be purchased for educational, business, or promotional use. For information on bulk purchases, please contact Macmillan Corporate and Premium Sales Department at 1-800-221-7945, extension 5442, or write specialmarkets@macmillan.com.

First Edition: May 2014

10 9 8 7 6 5 4 3 2

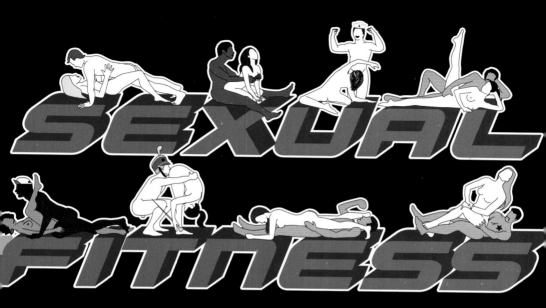

SEXUAL FITNESS

THE ULTIMATE GUIDE TO PUMP WHILE YOU HUMP, TONE WHILE YOU BONE AND SHRED IN THE BED

. Gugenheim, Marc Fellner-Erez, Anat Erez-Fellner and Lee Ash

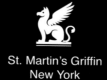

St. Martin's Griffin
New York

INTRO

Thank you for picking up SEXUAL FITNESS. We are excited to give you some guidance on a fun-filled journey. While we tried to make this book as entertaining as hell, we also strive to give you an incredible and ass-kicking challenge. The most important growth in life happens not just in your pants, but also when we push ourselves to venture outside of our comfort zone. With SEXUAL FITNESS we start outside some people's comfort zone – the erogenous zone! – and then we push you to the next level. What you and your lover are capable of achieving when you work this way should blow your mind! Boom.

Experts say that during a sexual romp the average person will burn between 100-150 calories. While there is no way of truly aggregating what you'll burn, the workouts we provide in SEXUAL FITNESS, when done correctly, are designed to help you burn between 220-400 calories per workout or more! That's huge! With the help of this book you should be able to take your sex life and your health to exciting new places. Yeah, we are excited for you.

Each workout is designed to engage as much of your body as possible and will allow you to go as fast or as slow and as hard or as soft as you wish. We will continue to remind you to flex and engage your core and other muscles, but you should always be focusing on building your strength by increasing the blood flow to all your muscles, not just your genitals! Spend time as a couple, have more fun while you bone, and get in great shape all at the same time! Go SEXUAL FITNESSIZE yourself!

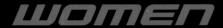

WOMEN

Hello, you strong, sexy, confident woman living in this fast-paced world. One key to modern survival is finding a balance in all the chaos. Many women enjoying taking yoga, Pilates or going to the gym to help balance their mind and tone their bod. Can't fit that in your busy schedule? SEXUAL FITNESS will fix that. We bring some of what would be learned in class right to your bedroom, your shower, your laundry room, really just about any-where that you can get away with it. When making your way through the orgasm-inducing workouts in this book you may choose to skip over any pose that you are not fully comfortable with. That's just fine. Communicate your desires to your partner. Try to let yourself go and take your sex life to new heights. Keep your mind and your legs open and enjoy the ride, girl!

MEN

Hey fella, welcome to the best workout ever. You may feel like a world-class porn star bodybuilder when you are mastering each pose, but remember the subtleties of lovemaking. There is a time and a place for the blasting jackhammer but use it with discretion. The aim is to be in control. That is how you get the most out of this book, sexually and physi-cally. Remember to communicate and connect with your body as well as your partner's body. Prematurely blowing your load will never be an issue because you will have the focus of mind and body to overcome the urge to cum. With the new confidence you gain from SEXUAL FITNESS you will enjoy all aspects of your life even more, both in and out of the bedroom. Oh, did we mention that you will have sex? Lots o' sex!

THE 10 COMMANDMENTS OF SEXUAL FITNESS

1	Thou shalt not hold your breath while exercising.
2	Listen to your partner's cues and stay in sync.
3	Engage your core throughout the workout.
4	Feel one another sensually and emotionally as well as physically.
5	Push your sexual limits.
6	Do not judge yourself or your partner.
7	Eat right.
8	Make a sex plan and follow through.
9	Communicate your desires.
10	Make it fun! Enjoy!!!

HOW TO GET WHAT WE GIVE - AKA MENU

These pages are designed to help you understand and navigate your way through this book. Check it out to see what all the different colors represent. Don't just look at the naked pictures, remember this is for your health. Don't worry, we'll get to the sex part right after this....

ILLUSTRATION

- Red is the primary muscle(s) being worked.

- Blue is the secondary muscle(s) being worked.

- Green is the muscle(s) being stretched.

WHO?

The pages are color coded to indicate what is being targeted in that particular pose.

STRETCH	HIM	HER	BOTH

TIPSY

All the exercise tips you need to know to get the most satisfaction out of each pose. You'll see the TIPSY on every page – use it.

MUSCLE CHART

This box names and ranks the muscles being exercised.

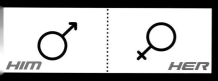

HIM | HER

HEY, DUDE, YOU KNOW WHICH ONE IS THE GUY? THE CIRCLE WITH THE BONER.

TICKER

This ticker indicates by color how difficult the position is. It will also suggest additional workouts to take your fitness to the next level.

>>> **EASY : FOREPLAY**

>>> **MODERATE : GETTING HOT**

>>> **HARD : HARD CORE**

>>> **EXTREME : CIRQUE DU FUCK**

DISCLAIMER

Attempt all activities in this book at your own risk.
The authors of Sexual Fitness are not responsible for any personal injury or damage to any property of any kind.

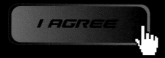

I AGREE

MUSCLE GUIDE

- **TRAPEZIUS - NECK/SHOULDERS**

- **DELTOID - SHOULDERS**

- **BICEP BRACHII - BICEPS, GUNS**

- **PECTORALIS MAJOR - PECS**

- **EXTERNAL OBLIQUE - SIDES**

- **EXTENSOR - FOREARMS**

- **RECTUS ABDOMINUS - ABS**

- **ABDUCTOR LONGUS - GROIN, INNER THIGHS, HIP FLEXORS**

- **GASTROCNEMIUS - CALVES**

- **RECTUS FEMORUS - QUADRICEPS, QUADS**

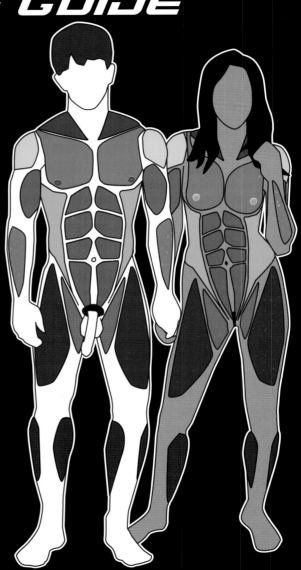

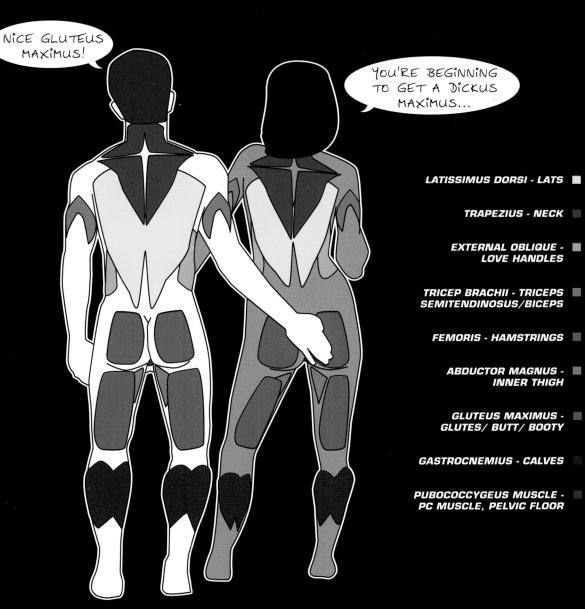

POSITIONS

FOREPLAY

GETTING HOT

HARD-CORE

CIRQUE DU FUCK

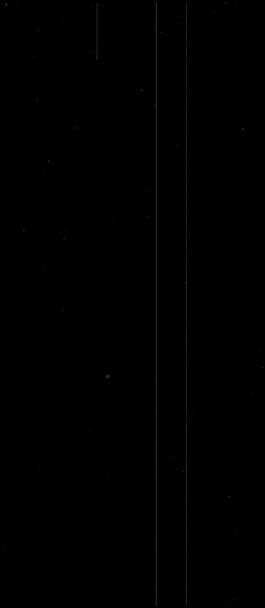

Always start with *FOREPLAY*
No matter how hot you think you are everyone needs to warm up!

7

A MAN A HAND A PLAN

You have the place to yourself, but you have to pace yourself. Think of it as a training session opportunity, engage your muscles and go slow. As you will see most of these poses are for couples. If you don't have a partner, boy, we ripped you off (now skip to Pose 68). For a more advanced workout replace hand with an actual female and get much more bounce to the ounce.

*also called: Beef Stroking Off, Choking the Chicken, Beating the Meat, Wanking It.

TIPSY

Resist the urge to cum. Stop yourself by using the strength of your pc muscle (located between your balls and your anus) as this will lead to longer-lasting bedroom blasting.

Drugs, alcohol, video games and remote controls are antithesis of Sexual Fitness.

For a better performance replace these vices/devices with vitamins, a balanced diet, healthy sleep, regular exercise and social activity.

Challenge yourself by using the weaker arm.

>>> BY DOING SIMPLE TOE RAISES DURING A SPANK SESSION YOU WILL INCREASE THE GIRTH OF YOUR DON

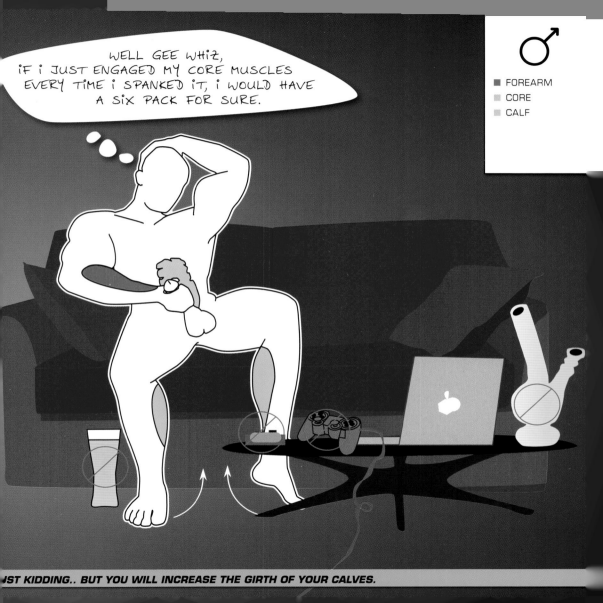

2

V FOR VAGINA*

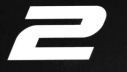

Sitting with her legs raised and her feet spread wide, she uses her fingers to bring herself to an amazing climax while working her lower body and core. If she puts her legs up flat against the wall it changes the workout into a great lower body stretch.

*AKA: Beating Around the Bush, Dousing the Digits, Muffin Buffin, Spelunking, Teasing the Taco.

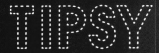

Remove your rings and trim your nails before trying this pose.

Turn your partner on by letting him watch you work it the way you want it (feel free to fantasize about whomever you want).

>>> IF YOU WANT TO DO IT STANDING UP JUST PUT A SLIGHT BEND IN YOUR KNEES AND WORK THOSE UPPI

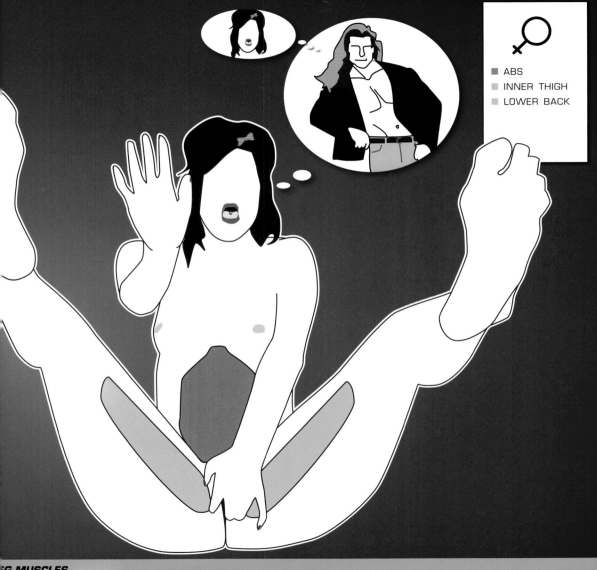

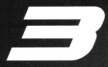

3

STRETCHERCISE

Sitting on the floor facing each other, both partners spread their legs and clasp their hands. Alternate gently pulling each other forward and holding the stretch for at least 10 seconds each time. The person who is pulling will get a little muscle warm-up while the one being pulled gets a nice easy stretch.

TIPSY

While warming up your bod try to reach your partner's genitals. Incentive for both people. Even if you don't reach, you get a great view and maybe a whiff of your partner's pheromones. The scent increases your heart rate, upping your level of arousal and warming your body simultaneously.

Stretch upwards and elongate your spine before folding over your legs for a healthier stretch.

>>> **THIS IS A GREAT STRETCH TO COUNTER THE SPHINXTER (POSE 14).**

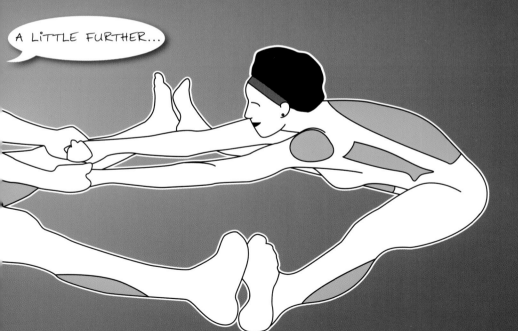

4
POWER LUNCH

She puts one leg up on a chair, a bed or whatever she can get her foot on and leans forward into a deep lunge. He lunches on her munch while she enjoys her stretch.

TIPSY

Her — Keep your feet facing forward, your core engaged, your lower back straight and your knee above your ankle. Enjoy.

Him — Hold on to her thighs so you can really get in there.

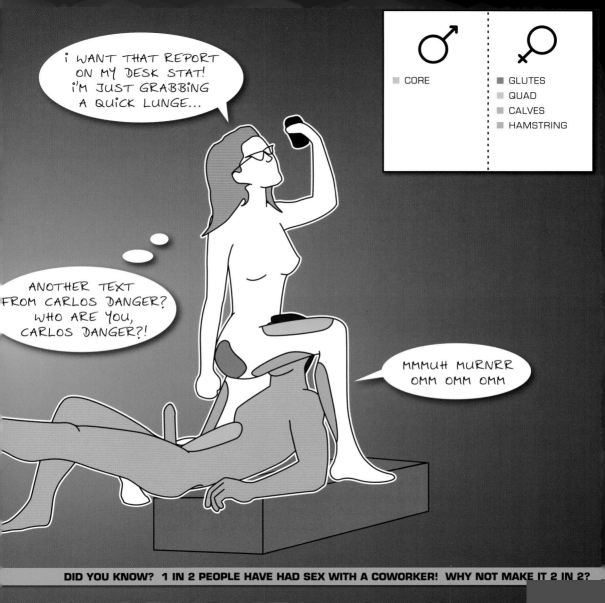

5
PARALLEL PARKING

Lying parallel, side by side, she raises her top leg to a 90-degree angle. He supports her from behind while his fingers gently titillate the tender petals of her labia and tickle her clitoris. He does leg lifts with his bottom leg for his own workout.

TIPSY

Her — Engage your core and keep your hips aligned with the rest of your body. Make sure to not rock forward or backwards. Slowly raise your leg by engaging your lower abs and glutes, then slightly lower it while engaging your hamstring. Repeat 30 times on each side.

If you need a break from those leg lifts you can use your Kegel muscle to squeeze his fingers inside you.

Him — Pleasure your woman, man! This one is all about her. Oh… and don't forget to whisper in her ear how great she is.

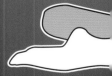

>>> FOR AN ADDED LEG WORKOUT SHE SHOULD ALTERNATE BETWEEN FLEXING AND POINTING HER TOES

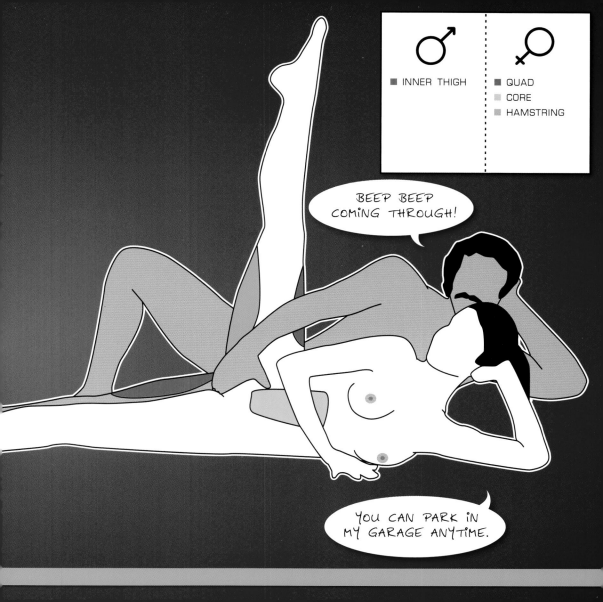

A HEAD START

Oral sex is a great time to multitask. No, don't check your email when your partner isn't looking and his or her mouth is full. Instead, shred while you get head.

TIPSY

For the giver — Plank, push-ups, leg lifts.

For the receiver — Perform crunches while getting pleasured by isolating and holding your body off the ground by engaging your core. Hold a medicine ball or a similarly heavy object in your hands and while reaching up towards the sky rotate your trunk left to right, engaging your obliques as you twist from side to side.

IF PLANK OR PUSH-UPS ARE TOO HARD WITH STRAIGHT LEGS, DO THEM WITH YOUR KNEES ON THE GROUND

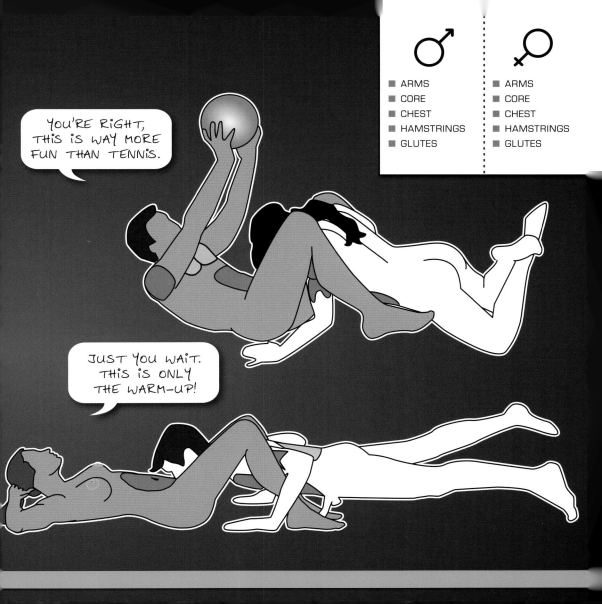

7
THE MERMAID AND THE SAILOR

From his knees he isometrically flexes his muscles. She balances by bending one knee in front of her and one behind her. Raising one arm above her head, she folds her body in the opposite direction as far as she can maintain, then repeats on the other side. If she likes what she sees, she may decide to pleasure his thingumabob, even though she has 20, who cares... she wants more.

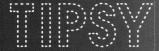

Her — Stretch up first and then over and do not collapse your rib cage. Use your bottom arm for support and stretch all the way through the upper arm.

Him — If you flex your body from this position you'll sustain an even harder and longer-lasting erection to let her fully enjoy her stretch. Dip your dick in the ocean and get it wet if you know what we mean....

>>> GREAT FOREPLAY POSE! GETTING YOU READY FOR ACTION!

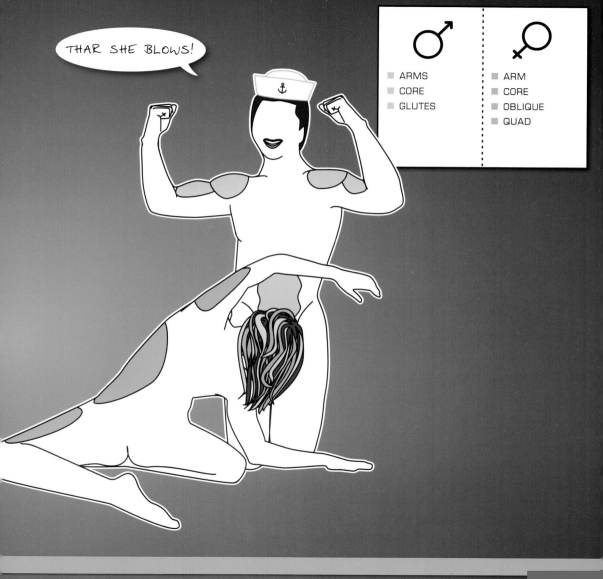

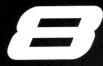

8

THE SQUATTING TROMBONER*

This one time, at Band Camp, she folded over with a flat back and touched her toes. He sustained a deep squat while blowing her mind from behind.

*also called: Smooching the Starfish.

TIPSY

Her — If you cannot reach your toes just rest your hands on your shins. Do not hold tension in your neck. Oh, when the saints go marching in your back door, just let it go. Tooting your tuba might ruin the tune.

Him — If you have no musical experience just imagine you are sitting back in a chair eating a delicious dripping ice cream cone while inflating a balloon. Breathe through your nose.

>>> *THE DEEPER SHE LEANS FORWARD, THE MORE HE CAN PLEASURE HER.*

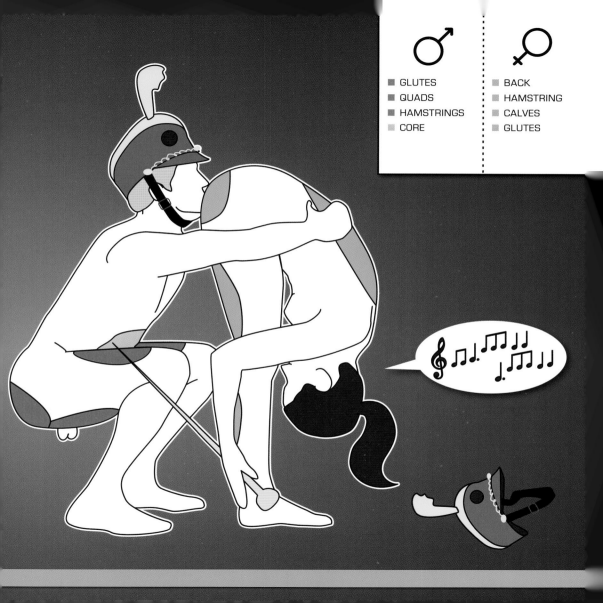

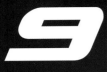

MISSIONARY POSITION

The woman lies on her back and beckons her man. The man braces himself on his hands and enters her pink cathedral from above.

*also called: The Matrimonial Position, The Mama-Papa Position and The English-American Position.

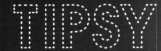

WHAT!

Her - You can engage your abs even more by raising your feet 6 inches. Tuck your tailbone to increase G-spot stimulation. Use a pillow for lower back support.

Him - Be on your hands instead of your elbows. Keep your knees off the bed. These two little adjustments will change this common pose to your favorite new exercise.

>>> ALTERNATE BETWEEN PUSH-UP AND FOREARM POSITION AND REDISTRIBUTE YOUR WEIGHT REGULAR.

ARMS
CHEST
ABS
LOWER BACK

GLUTES
ABS

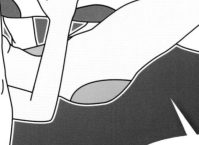

10
A MISSION WITH A TWIST

Your mission, if you choose to accept it, is to take the missionary position to the next level. The male undercover agent moves one leg to the outside of the female agent's legs and puts his weight on the opposite arm. He engages his obliques while thrusting from his core. This man will blow his load in 3…2…1…Sploog!

TIPSY

Her — Enjoy this position as his pubic bone has greater contact and friction with your clitoris. If you insist on a little exercise, which we totally appreciate, flex your tummy for a mild core workout. You're a woman of many parts.

Him — Use your free hand to pleasure her so you'll be forced to engage your lowered oblique. Work one side for 10 thrusts and switch arms. Enjoy her Pussy Galore.

>>> IF SHE WANTS A BETTER WORKOUT SHE SHOULD RAISE HER FEET 6 INCHES OFF THE BED.

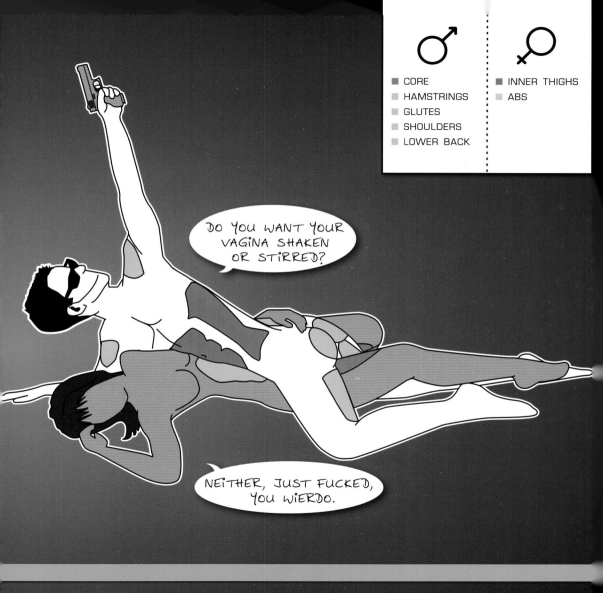

11

SLIGHTLY HARD-CORE

Already engaged in intercourse, with her body facing away from his, she moves into a plank position on her forearms while keeping his cock deep within her. She controls the tempo and intensity of the hump.

TIPSY

Her — If big movements prove problematic in this pose keep your body still and focus on working his dick through Kegel exercises.

Him — Engage your core and pull your pubic bone toward your stomach. You can support her by placing your hands on her sexy ass.

>>> BE WARY OF HIS ERECT MANHOOD AS IT IS FORCED DOWNWARD. YOU DON'T WANT TO BREAK IT.

12

SEXUAL INCLINATION*

Starting from reverse cowgirl (pose 34) she lowers her chest toward the bed, allows her knees to touch the bed, and does push-ups. He lies on his back and points his dick toward his toes.

*also called: The Fucking Female Push-Up, You Gotta Push Up to Get Down.

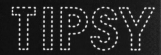

Her — Keep your core engaged to protect your back. The closer together you place your hands, the more you work out your triceps. The farther apart you place your hands, the more you work out your chest. Try to get your humps in rhythm with your pumps, uh - push-ups.

Him — Enjoy watching her take control. You can always give her a nice butt rub to get her going!

>>> *FOR MORE ADVANCED, SHE CAN DISTRIBUTE HER WEIGHT TO HER TOES INSTEAD OF HER KNEES.*

13

FANTASY LAND

Everyone has a character that they fantasize about. One that your partner would even let you smurf if the opportunity presented itself. So make your dreams cum true, close your eyes. Keep your hands, feet and erection inside the moving vehicle at all times and enjoy the ride. Make it matterhorny, next stop, huge splash mountain.

TIPSY

Her — Engage your legs, core and arms to rock your body up and down. Control the pace and enjoy the unique angle of penetration.

Him — Sit up on your sit bone using your abs to support your straight back. Your knees may need to be bent in order to keep your upright posture. Focus on your abdominal isolation as she rides you fast.

>>> IF HER LEGS GET TIRED SHE CAN ARCH HER BACK FOR A NICE BACK STRETCH.

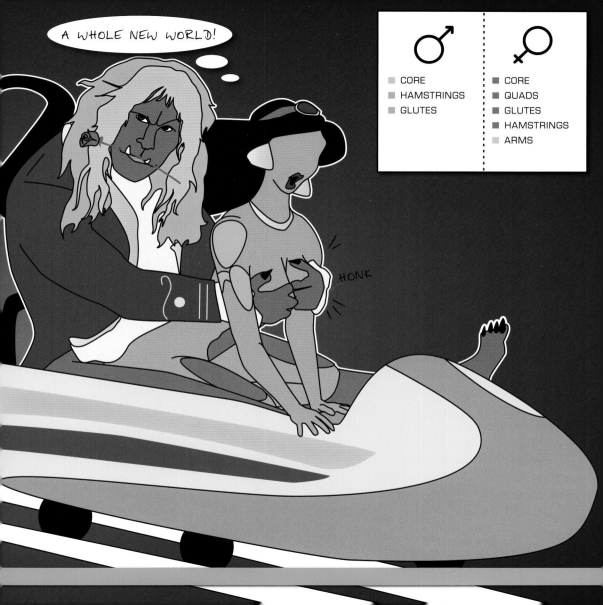

14

THE SPHINXTER

He finds himself crawling through the desert, parched, dizzy, starved for a drink and then off in the distance he sees a beautiful oasis. A lush watering hole.

TIPSY

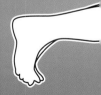

Her — Tighten your glutes and press up with your arms shining your heart forward with an open chest. Your head should be an extension of the spine, resting atop your neck with no crunching of your spine.

Him — You can switch to plank position on your elbows so you can use your hands to pry apart her cheeks and get in there.

Both — Sex is like a fountain of youth because it actually increases your life span.

>>> *WHILE IN PLANK HE CAN ALTERNATE LIFTING A FULLY POINTED AND EXTENDED LEG OFF THE GROUND.*

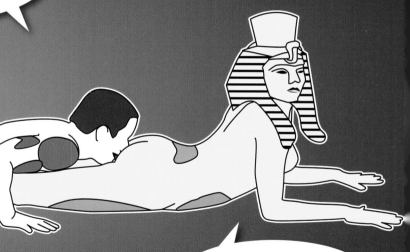

15
THE PELVIC THRUST

Every girl is crazy for a semi-dressed man, and vice versa. Buy a new outfit, get a hotel room and get it on like you are meant to. She straddles him with one of her legs between his legs. Using his abs, he lifts one leg to 45 degrees and the other leg is bent with his knee pointing to the sky.

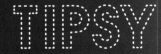

Her — Tighten your core. You can do single-handed tricep dips using his shoulder or bed for support.

Him — Thrust as high as you can ten times. That is one set. Do six sets on each side. If you get tired, she can stretch your groin, glutes, and quads. Take the time to work both legs and to get her off.

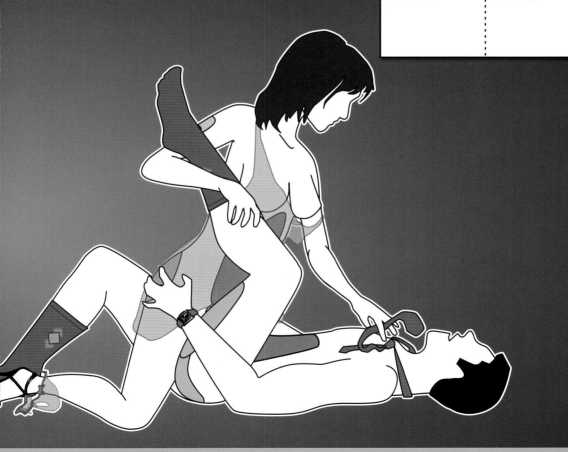

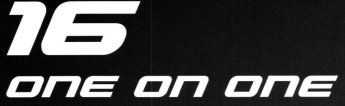

16
ONE ON ONE

In this pick-up game you play with 2 balls. Using her abs, she lifts one leg to 45 degrees and the other leg is extended on the floor or bed. He straddles her with one of his legs between her legs.

OH HONEY, YOUR WOODY IS MUCH BIGGER. BESIDES, WHITE MEN CAN'T HUMP.

TIPSY

Her — Activate your arm muscles by pressing your straight arms onto the floor or bed.

Him — Do push ups or isolate your chest by pressing into the floor or bed. Initiate your thrust using your lower abs. Take it to the hole.

>>> IN ADDITION TO ALTERNATING BETWEEN LEGS SHE CAN RAISE BOTH LEGS, ALLOWING HIM TO PLUNGE DEE

♂	♀
▪ TRICEPS	▪ ABS
▪ CORE	▪ HAMSTRING
▪ LOWER BACK	▪ GLUTES
▪ GLUTES	

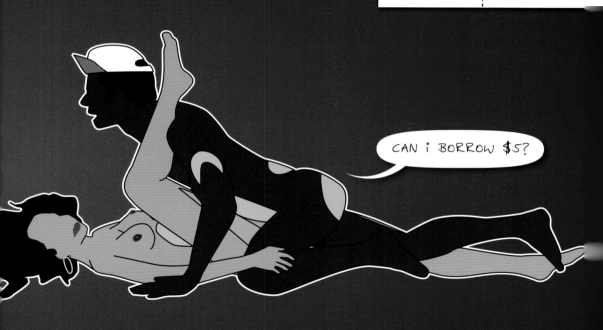

CAN i BORROW $5?

HILE INCREASING HER HAMSTRING STRETCH.

17

SYNCHRONIZED SCREWING

If sex was an Olympic sport this could be your chance. These two athletes may not appear to be doing much but the slow movements done as one body can stimulate the whole self and put the mind in a trancelike state of arousal.

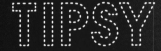

Her — Make sure your core is fully engaged as you lean back and then pull upwards again. Ride him in between crunches to heighten your enjoyment and prolong your abdominal sculpting.

Him — Rock your pelvis softly by tightening and curving your core. Then give her a little help by pushing her upwards with your chest against her back while flexing your core. Keep your dick in her box.

Both — Allow whatever happens to happen. Get in sync.

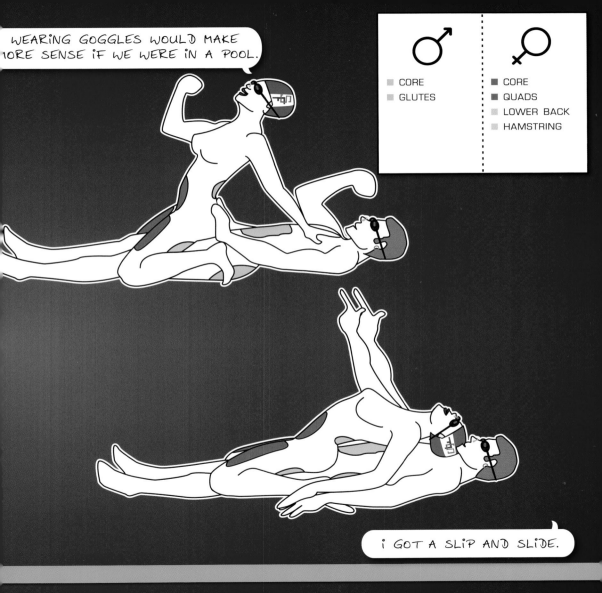

TWIST AND SPOUT

Move the G-string and stretch that hamstring. The Twist is a huge part of this workout. Make sure to always come back to center before each twist and switch the arm that is extended. The key here is to not stop thrusting. Come up with a rhythm: thrust, thrust, thrust, twist left, "uh, uh," thrust, thrust, thrust, twist center, "oh yeah," thrust, thrust, thrust, twist right, "omigod," thrust, thrust, thrust, twist center... and so on.

TIPSY

Her — Every time he twists, stretch to the opposite leg. (Note: G-strings are not necessary for this position to work out your muscles, they are just an added bonus.)

Him — Flex your abs every time you twist and breathe out all your air. Breathe back in slowly when you return to neutral. Alternate between a hard bicep flex and a fully extended arm on both sides. This makes you look very sexy.

LOWER BACK MUSCLES MAKE YOU LOOK LIKE A GREEK GOD! IT'S BAD ASS SO DON'T COMPROMISE FORM

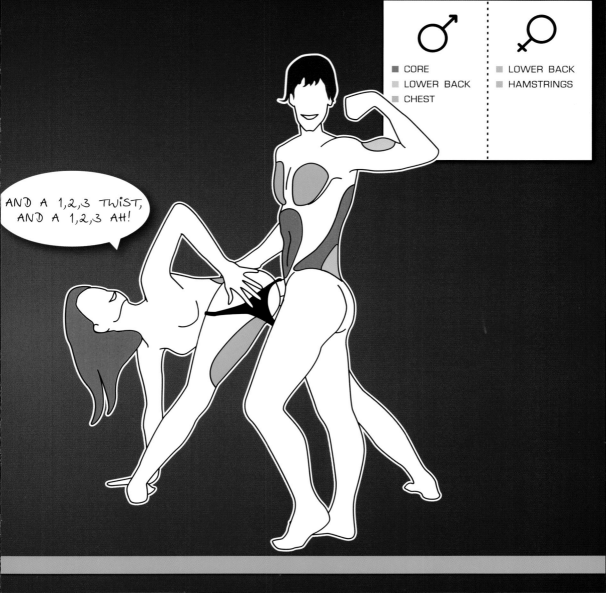

19

THE PIZZA BOY'S TIP

She orders a large sausage pie and curls up on the edge of the bed awaiting the delivery in a comfortable child's pose with her arms extended in front of her or down by her sides. He arrives to find the front door open and Sade pulsing from the stereo. He approaches the bed and enters her from behind, gently pushing her into a deeper stretch. He cums in 30 minutes or more, or it's free. It's her turn for a big tip.

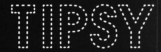

Her — The standard child's pose is with your arms extended above your head, but feel free to adapt it and bring your hands down, fondling his balls.

Him — The more you keep your core muscles engaged, the more you'll be able to maximize this simple position. Remember to scoop your core inwards and upwards to shred the lower abs and give her something to really enjoy.

>>> *TO INCREASE THE WORKOUT SHE CAN ENGAGE HER ARMS WITH SIMPLE PUSH-UPS.*

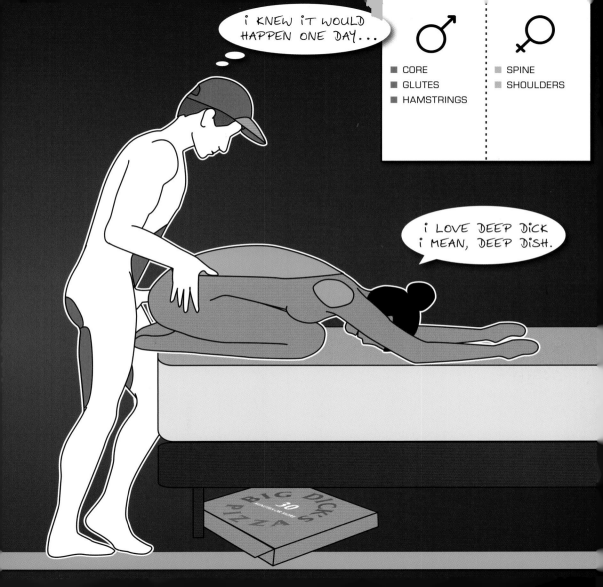

THE SNAKE CHARMER

You may feel like it is a day at the zoo with so many animals running around. She starts in tabletop position on a tabletop, his snake slithers in from behind, and she begins rolling between a cat and cow stretch. Get hypnotized as you cycle through all the incarnations. Become a sex animal.

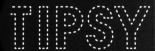

TIPSY

Her — Breathe nice and deep in perfect rhythm with the rise and fall of your body. Use his snake to explore your cave and discover your most pleasurable nooks and crannies.

Him — To get more of a leg workout you should stand on tippy toes to work your calves or bend your knees into a squat to work those quads. Do not let your snake bite her or she might bite it back.

BREAK OUT THAT PUNGI AND GET HYPNOTIC.

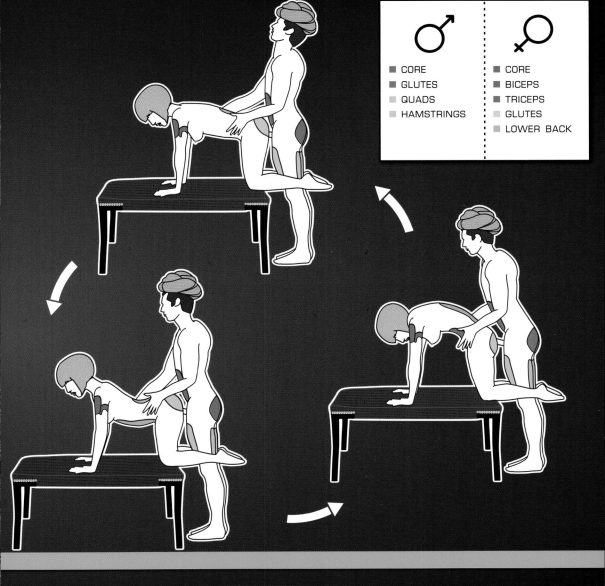

♂ CORE
■ GLUTES
■ QUADS
■ HAMSTRINGS

♀ CORE
■ BICEPS
■ TRICEPS
■ GLUTES
■ LOWER BACK

21
DOGGY STYLE

She is on her hands and knees. Gripping her hips, he slips her a bone. Then the bass kicks in. 1, 2, 3 and to the fo', looks like the little lady let the doggy in the back do'.

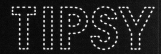

TIPSY

Her — For a harder arm workout, reach back and fondle his balls.

If you bend an arm into a half push-up you will double the chest workout. You can also do a full push-up for a more intense core workout.

Him — Reach around and stimulate her clit for a good stretch in the back and forearm. We don't recommend calling her a bitch. Fo' rizzeal.

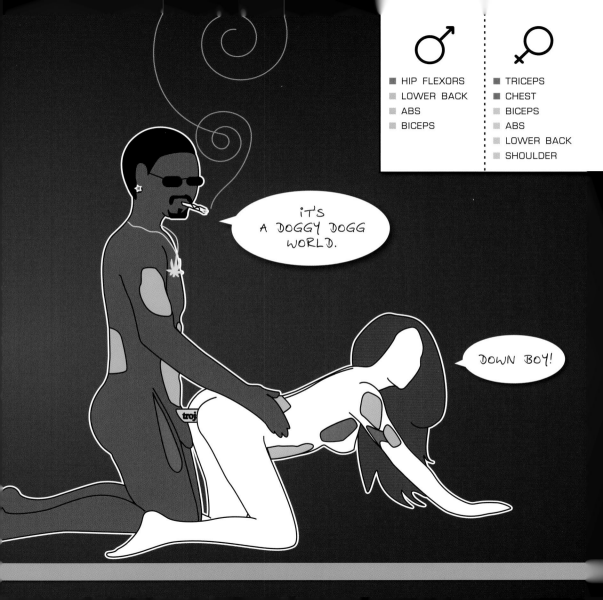

22
SEXRATARY*

She bends over the desk. He enters her from behind in professional appropriate manner. Monday just got a whole lot better.

*also called: Business and Pleasure, Tempting the Temp, Punching the Time Card.

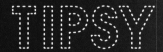

Her — As you lean over, keep a flat back by engaging your abs. You can deepen the workout by pushing up through your arms to work your pecs, and upper back. Pretend you are still wearing your high heels to tone those calves.

Him — If she's been naughty, give her a light spanking. Keep your muscles flexed to get them shredded in even the simplest positions. Don't just pump your thrust, make sure to scoop your core inwards and upwards.

>>> SHE CAN DO SEMI-SQUATS, WHICH WORK DIFFERENT MUSCLES AND GIVE DIFFERENT SENSATIONS TO BOT

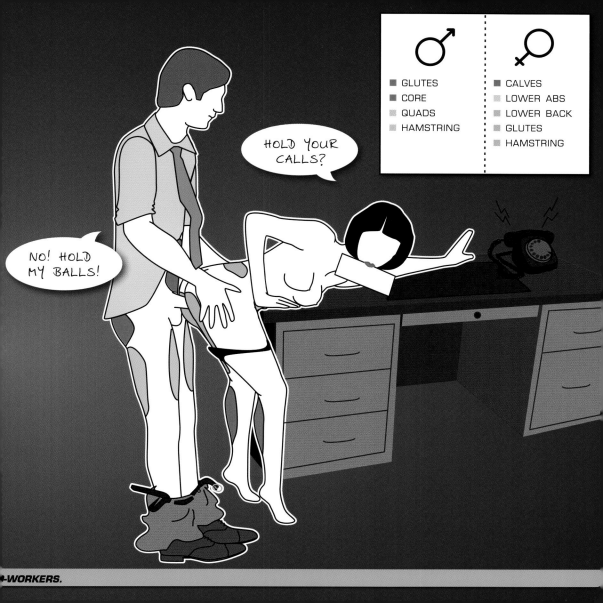

It's *GETTING HOT* in here....

23
CUNNILINGUS*

The cunning linguist is a master at fulfilling this pose
Trilling his tongue as he peddles his prose
To a sexy young thing who hears it and knows
She can command where that talented tongue goes

*AKA: Nursin' the Curtains, The Michael Douglas.

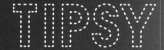

Her — Bend towards the floor until you feel a good stretch you can maintain. Do a child's pose (pose 19) afterwards to counter the stretch. You don't want to compress your lower spine or strain your neck.

Him — Raising your feet 6 inches off the bed will work your abs. For a stretch, place the soles of your feet together and let your legs fall apart so they form a diamond shape. Romance always works.

>>> *NOW IT'S HIS TURN TO STRETCH WHILE YOU LICK HIS BALLS.*

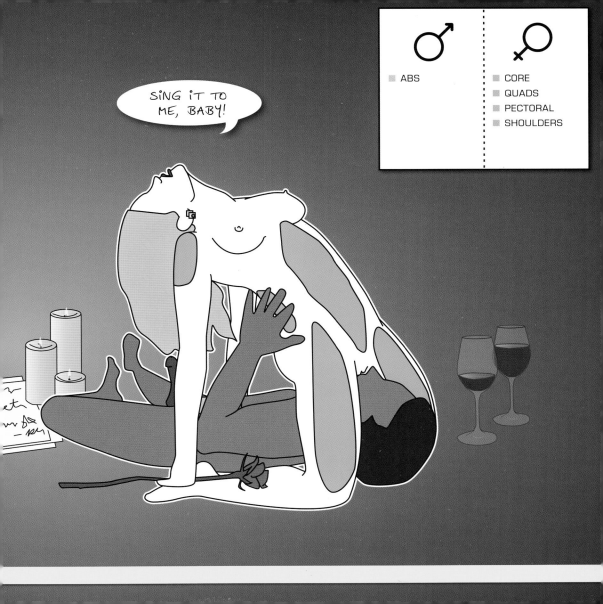

24

TAKING 69 UP A NOTCH

She lies on her back, performs a bridge, and then lifts one leg up as far as she can. He gets on all fours, starting with a neutral spine, then performs alternating cat to cow. While pleasuring each other they switch every 30 seconds, him from cat to cow and her between raised legs.

TIPSY

Her — Keep your core tight to protect your back. Don't put pressure on your neck. Keep your leg straight. Better that the leg is not all the way up than if it bends. Work on bringing the straight leg back by engaging your lower abs and glutes.

Him — You can upside down titty-fuck her while she licks your taint. Sweet!

>>> SHE CAN FLEX AND POINT HER RAISED FOOT AND DO SMALL ANKLE CIRCLES.

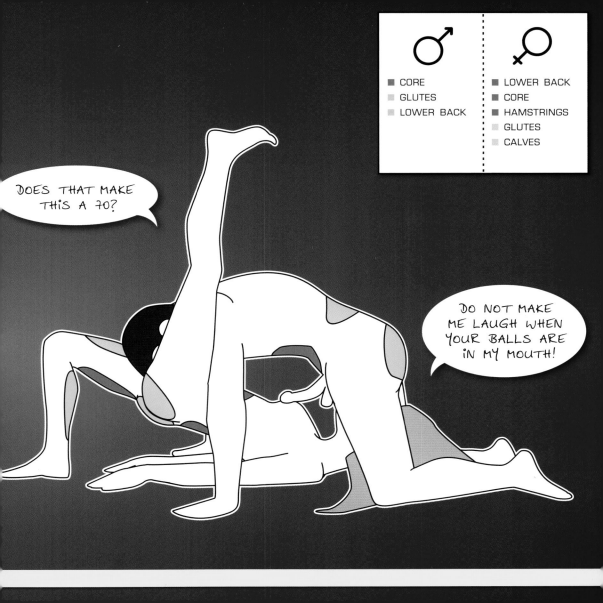

25

THE PINK DIAMOND

While everyone knows that skiing is when a lady jerks off two dudes at the same time, just imagine something more personal and romantic. After a few warm beverages you leave the lodge of your alpine resort and head toward your room. The snow is falling outside your window. You are amped to hit the slopes the next morning at 6 a.m. but tonight is your chance to work on your form. Pretend you are skiing and he is sledding and go to town, naked. Not recommended for actual use on the slopes.

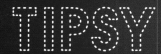

Her — Keep your form and enjoy his warm mouth. Give him the Peek-a-boo stance.

Him — Lean back on your elbows to support your core and focus on pleasing your woman. A single pink diamond is worth 10 blue squares. Wear lip balm to avoid chapping.

Both — Beware of cold weather, it can cause shrinkage and permafrost nips. Watch out for avalanches.

>>> HE CAN ALLEVIATE WEIGHT FROM HER BODY BY USING HIS HANDS TO PUSH UP ON HER GLUTES WH

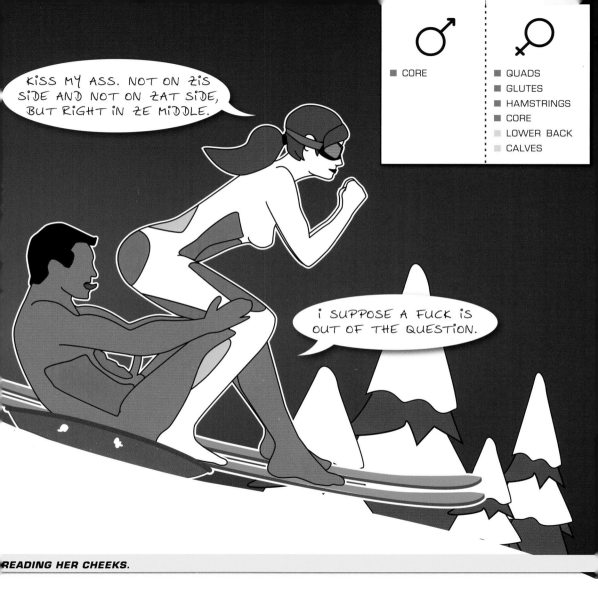

26
THE CARROT ON A STRING

Sometimes people need a little encouragement.... From a flat position on the floor, she raises her legs and chest simultaneously while he does squats. The trick is to time this out so she gets her head to his crotch while he is at the right depth of squat. Give a kiss and relax. Engage again.

TIPSY

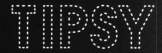

Her — Engage your core to protect your lower back while achieving the V. If you can't raise your legs, try to keep them bent parallel to the floor. If you need more incentive semen is an anti-aging agent that has a tightening effect on the skin.

Him — Sit back in an imaginary chair. Careful not to put too much pressure on your knees as they want to be directly in line with your ankles. You want your quads to do most of the work.

>>> **THIS CAN BE REPEATED BY REVERSING THE ROLES.**

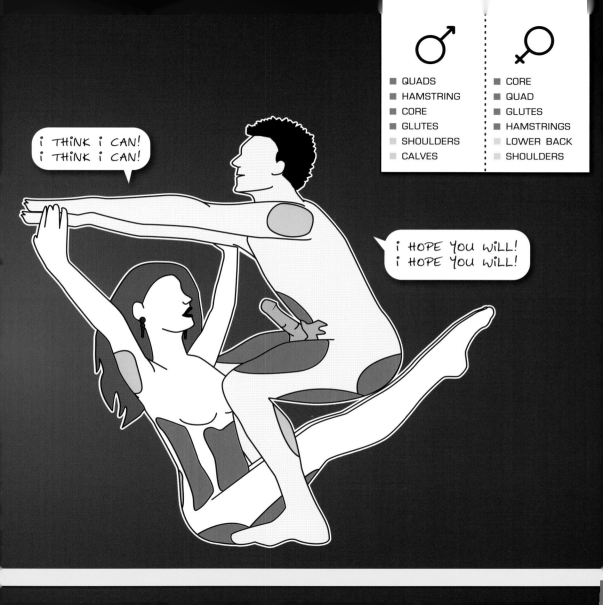

27
THE SEA LION

The male sea lion dives deep into the kelp forest of love. Playfully and not in any hurry the female sea lion raises her legs up into the air and sets them on the male's shoulders. The two experience the motion of the ocean.

OH YEAH, FUCK ME LIKE A SEA LION.

TIPSY

Her — You can move into a raised split for an inner thigh stretch. This will also elongate and tighten the inside of your vagina.

Him — Get off your knees and get into an angled plank position for an abdominal workout.

Both - For deep stimulation you should focus on scooping your lower core towards each other instead of thrusting.

>>> SHE CAN DO PELVIC THRUSTS AGAINST HIS PUMPS TO INCREASE HER WORKOUT.

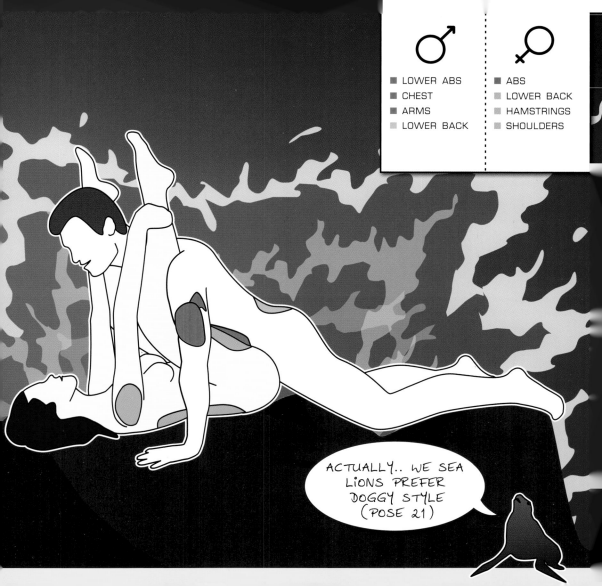

28

THE BALLERINA BUNNIES

She lies on her back and, engaging her abs, raises her legs and spreads them like bunny ears. He tickles the space between. This bunny is hotter than any in those magazines. Thumper, thumper hard.

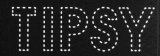

TIPSY

Her — The higher up you raise your legs the better a stretch it is for your spine. Keep your weight on your shoulder blades so you don't strain your neck. Concentrate on your breathing. You can support your lower back with your hands while you rest your elbows on the floor.

Him — Focus on pleasing her with your fingers or anything else that she likes. Or you can head down the rabbit hole. Keep your abs flexed as you focus.

Both — Sex toys can be added to almost any pose for those times you wish you had two Peters.

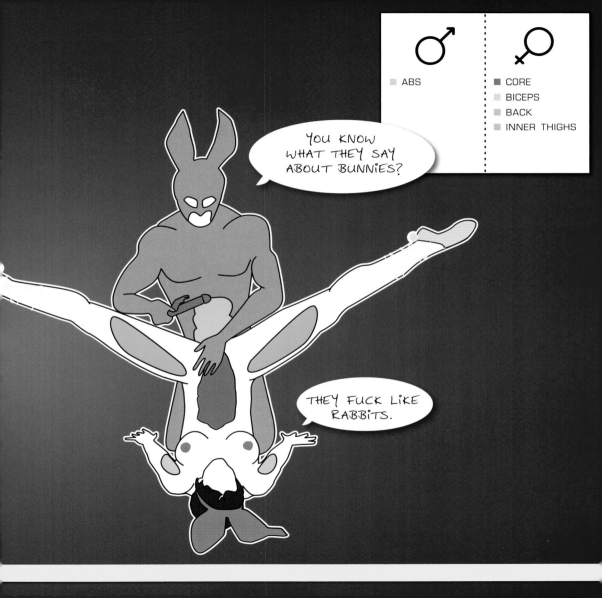

29
HEAD COACH

Even the best Sexual Fitness pros need a little coaching from time to time. He dips his bar as he does bar dips with one leg up. He is greatly rewarded for his efforts by his head cheerleader. Get your head in the game! He cheers on his girl and lets her know what it takes to reach his peak. Cum on team!

TIPSY

Her — Make it harder on him by applying your body weight. Engage your core as you push forward and backwards with your arms. You may want to use a pillow for your knees.

Him — Not only are you working your upper body with chest dips and isolations, but the added leg lifts get you the leg up on the competition.

TO INCREASE HER CORE WORKOUT SHE CAN PUT HER HANDS BEHIND HER BACK.

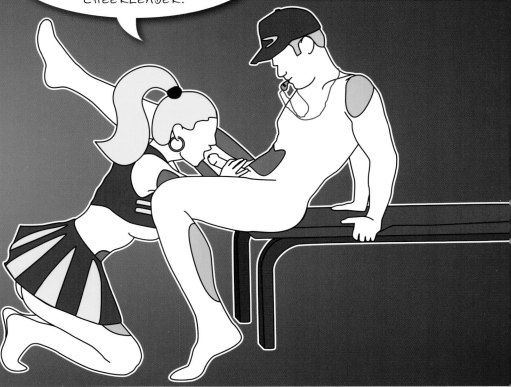

30

INVITE HIM UP AND TIE HIM DOWN

After a nice dinner and a show she invites him up for an encore performance. She ties him to the bed. Either facing him or facing away (so he doesn't see how hard she's working), she slides him into her cookie as she lowers herself into a deep squat. From there she rides him by slightly lifting and lowering herself while engaged in the squat. Squats, camera, get some action!

TIPSY

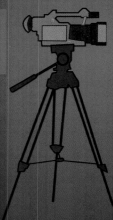

Her — Keep your core tight and don't forget to protect your knees.

Him — Put a large pillow under your ass to raise your hips so she doesn't have to go too low.

Both — Keep good track of where you store your sex vids. A leaked sex tape can ruin your career, or in the case of the Kardashians it can make your career. Find a safe word. We recommend "Anastasia."

>>> IF THE RESTRAINTS ARE STRONG HE CAN WORK HIS MUSCLES BY PULLING AGAINST THEM.

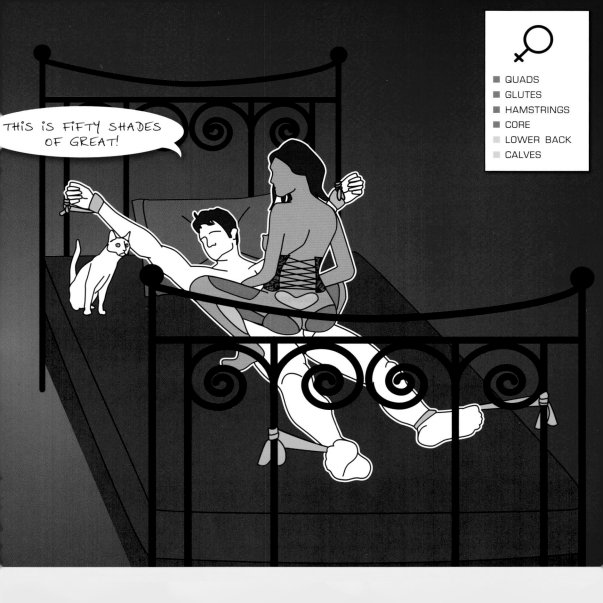

THE DIVINE STOMACH

Straddling the man, she leans back and gets a workout for her arms and upper back. He does too.

*also called: The Dueling Coyotes, The Double Bridge.

TIPSY

Her — If the stretch is too intense for you, rest your hands on his thighs and sit upright.

Him — Straighten legs for a different workout and angle of penetration.

Both — Use knee pads or a pillow to protect your joints. Stay focused on your partner even though you do not have direct eye contact. Do not let your mind wander.

>>> FOR HARD-CORE BOTH PARTNERS MOVE IN AND HOLD EACH OTHER FOR 30 SECONDS, FOR CIRQUE DU FU

SHE PLACES HER ANKLES ON HIS SHOULDERS.

32

THE LOTUS

With the man seated on the floor in a yogi-like meditation, the woman opens the delicate petals of her sexual flower and lowers herself upon his bow staff. They wrap their arms around one another and rock their way to nirvana.

TIPSY

Enjoy each other's warmth. This position is about connection and balance.

Rest your muscles by allowing your skeletal system to properly stack itself.

2 be cum 1.

BOTH PARTNERS SHOULD FLEX THEIR ENTIRE BODIES IN ORDER TO ATTAIN A WORKOUT.

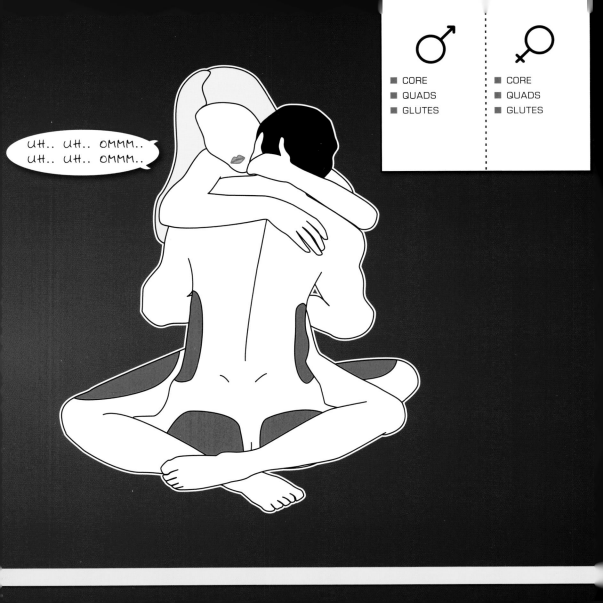

33

DOUBLE PLANK

Shiver me boner! It's a pirate's life for 2. Wenches be warned he may try to steal your booty. Starting from a position where he is inside her and on top of her backside they raise their bodies together. She gets into a low plank by distributing her weight on her forearms. He gets into a standard plank. From here they do an elevated horizontal hump and bump. If he is an ass pirate there may even be some action on the poop deck. Arrr you ready?!

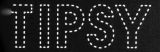

TIPSY

Her — Keep your core tight to hold your body straight. Use your lower abs and lower back muscles to pull your booty up and into him. The tighter you hold your core the better your workout. He will probably need assistance in removing your corset because of his hook hand.

Him — Use your lower abs and lower back muscles to scoop and thrust and pleasure her. The tighter you hold your core the better your workout.
X marks the G-spot

IF BOTH FEEL STRONG, DISTRIBUTE YOUR WEIGHT TOWARD ONE SIDE AT A TIME FOR TEN COUNTS.

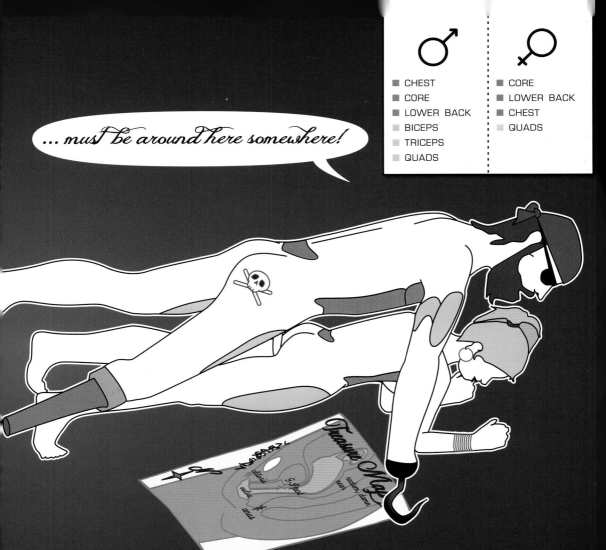

34

THE REVERSE COWGIRL*

This pose is great if you are at the beach and only have one towel or are in the desert and only have one bed roll, because it keeps the sand out of your stage cooch. With the man on his back she does sit-ups on his dick. Remember that sex on public beaches is outlawed. So be an outlaw.

*also called: Sex on the Beach.

TIPSY

Her — Keep your core engaged so you can lean back while you ride your stud.

Him — Keep your legs and upper body off the ground to increase your workout.

Both — For a great workout you can do leg lifts. Make sure to bring a towel unless you have two.

>>> SHE SHOULD NOT USE HER ARMS AS SUPPORT, THIS WILL GIVE HER A MORE INTENSE CORE WORKOUT.

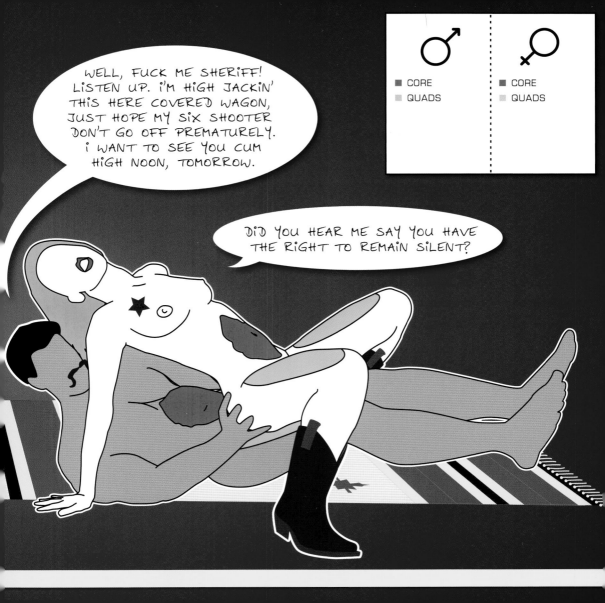

35

THE PILE DRIVER*

Lying on her back, she raises herself up by placing her heels onto his shoulders. Clutching her thighs, he drives his manhood deep into her silky folds. Coed naked wrestling is a fantastic aerobic workout.

*also called: Knockin' on the Back Door, The Anaconda Squeeze.

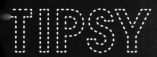

Her — Hold your abs tight and careful with your feet placement.

Him — You can hold her hands and do curls with her body weight.

TO TAKE IT TO THE NEXT LEVEL SHE CAN GRAB HIS WRISTS AND PULL HERSELF TO DO A VERTICAL SIT-UP.

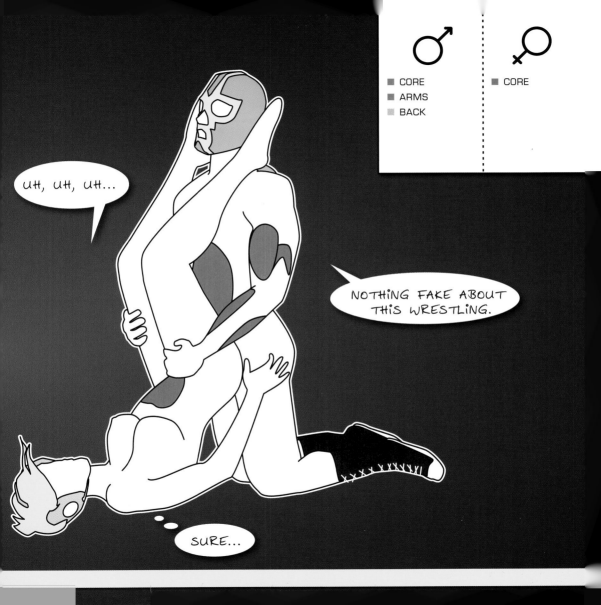

36

THE TUMBLER

She does a downward dog stretch and then places the crown of her head on a soft surface. Lifting her heels, she opens her loins to his impending love.

TIPSY

Her — Don't fall. Concentrate on your breathing and balance. Do your best to do little shoulder push-ups.

Him — Keep your core active and pulse your arms against her hips. You must be careful not to injure her head or neck!

>>> SHE SHOULD NOT STAY IN THIS POSITION TOO LONG OR SHE'LL GET A HEAD RUSH. GET UP SLOWLY.

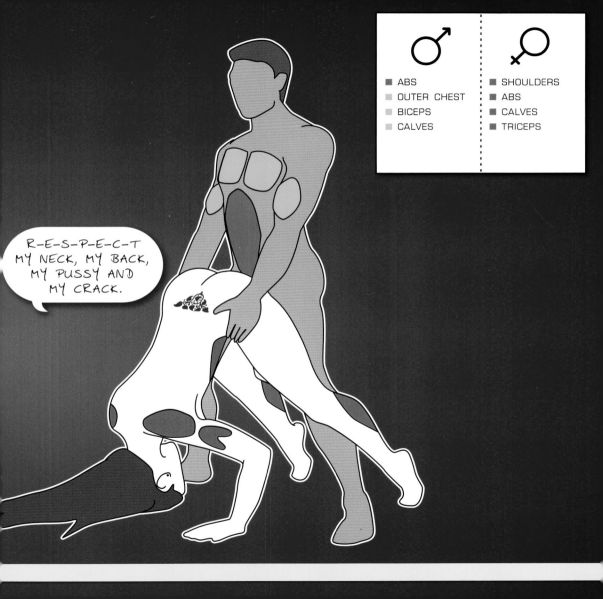

37

THE DIRTY DANCERS

Are you interested in having the time of your life? Experiencing feelings you never felt before? There is a healthy, sexy epidemic sweeping the nation. Pole-dancing for a workout, not just for filthy dolla bills. Get to a local pole-dancing class, heck, get a pole installed in your bedroom and get down. If you can't install a pole in your place, feel free to use your partner's pole or just dance around. It's a turn-on and a great workout.

TIPSY

Move to the groove. Be careful to focus on the different muscles you are engaging and stretching. Don't over-extend. She should be careful with her neck if she performs fellatio from downward dog. And he should be careful with his neck if he performs cunnilingus from a seated back bend.

In fact, everyone should be careful when dirty dancing. We can't tell you how many emergency room visits each year are attributed to pole-dancing injuries. Really, we can't.

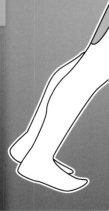

PUMP UP THE MUSIC, GET NAKED AND DANCE. WHAT A WILD FLASH MOB THIS WOULD BE!

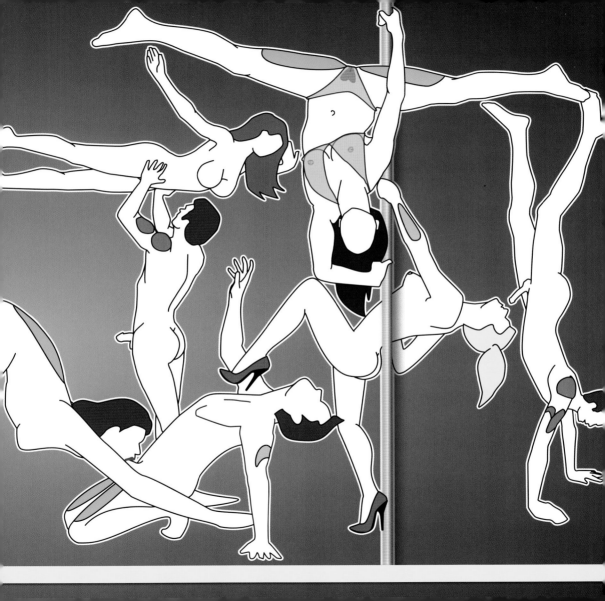

38
LEG UP DOGGY

From the classic Doggy Style (pose 21) he helps her lift one of her legs up and straight back over his thigh. Be careful not to get stuck.

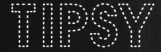

TIPSY

Her — Be sure to engage your core and not let your lower back sag. You are man's sexiest friend. If you would like to tone your arms and core even more you can do one-arm push-ups.

Him — Watch her carefully and support her. Pump softly and help her keep her balanced.

Both — Padded surfaces are your friends.

>>> IF YOU ARE BOTH UP FOR IT HE CAN RAISE HIMSELF INTO A MEDIUM-HIGH LUNGE BY RAISING THEIR KNE.

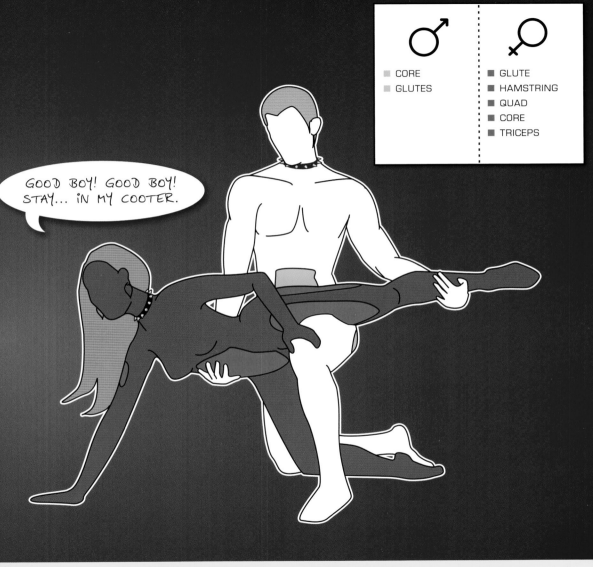

39

OH YES, DRILL SERGEANT

Alright, you maggots. I want him to grab some pole while she grabs the Private's privates. Both warriors work the shit out of their biceps until they can go no further, then they go a little further. He does pull-ups into her mouth while she strokes and throats his gun. Suck with pride and await his honorable discharge

TIPSY

Her — If he needs assistance you can put your hands on his ass and raise him up, easing the strain on him while working your back.

Him — If it gets to be too much just hang and pump your hips.

MAKE SURE YOUR COCK DOESN'T WRITE CHECKS YOUR MOJO CAN'T CASH.

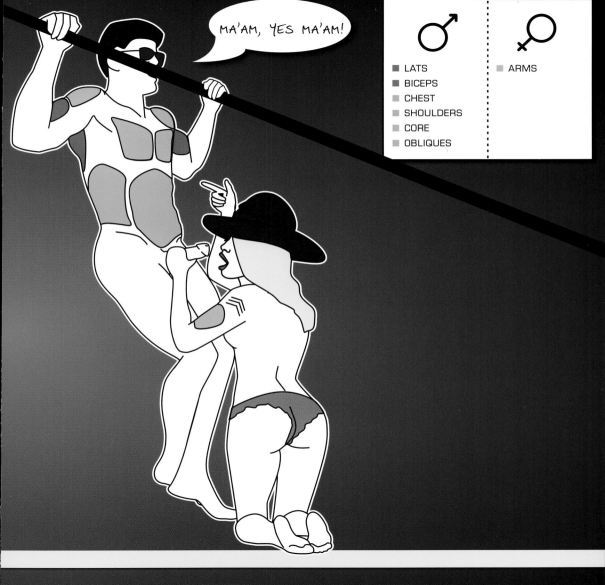

40
PRESS À TROIS

For the Sexual Fitness enthusiast who is ready for some serious heavy lifting or for the novice who needs incentive to hit the weights. Start by finding two sexy workout partners and head to your private gym. There he does bench presses while one woman rides his face and the other rides his dong. Then everyone rotate. Adjust the weight as needed and pump that pussy or rather, pump that iron.

*also called: The Jane Fonda.

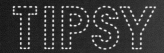

"[The Pump] as satisfying to me as cumming is, you know, as in having sex with a woman and cumming. So can you believe how much I am in heaven? I am like getting the feeling of cumming in the gym; I'm getting the feeling of cumming at home; I'm getting the feeling of cumming backstage; when I pump up, when I pose out in front of 5000 people I get the same feeling, so I am cumming day and night. It's terrific, right? So you know, I am in heaven."

Arnold Schwarzenegger - "Pumping Iron"

>>> *FOR HARD-CORE ENTHUSIASTS HE CAN LIFT HIS LEGS UP OFF THE FLOOR.*

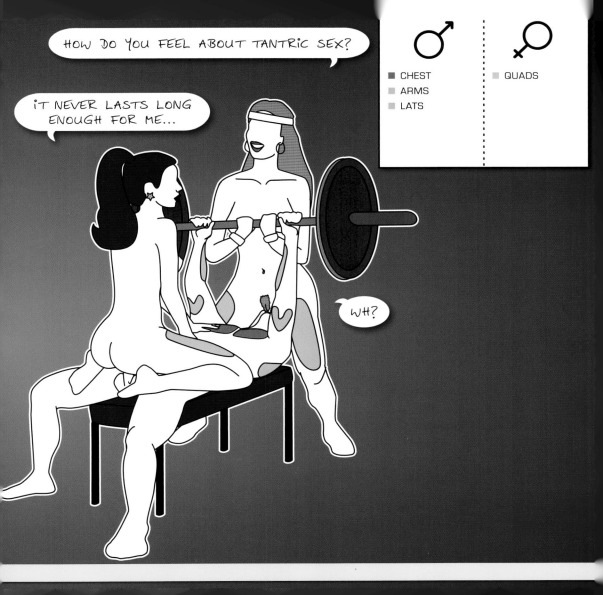

Screw PG-13, this is **HARD-CORE**

41

I DREAM OF CREAMING ON JEANNIE

The man is doing a shoulder stand while the woman jerks or sucks him off until all his wishes cum true. We recommend wearing costumes to get you in the mood.

TIPSY

Her — Please your Major! And revel in the satisfaction of him squealing as he climaxes to an altitude he previously thought impossible.

Him — Tuck in your chin so you can see what she is doing and protect your neck at the same time. Inverting your body increases circulation flowing back to the heart from the lower body. Better circulation equals sustained erections and a healthier heart!

Both — Beware when he climaxes. Safety goggles may be needed to avoid ejaculate fluid.

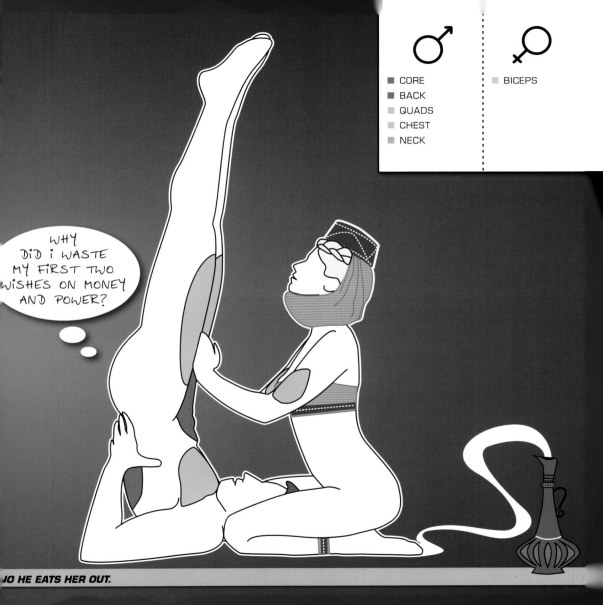

42

SHANKLAMBANKA*

After a few cold vodka shots these Russian dolls perform a traditional dance. She rolls back, exposing her sputnik, scooping her abs in and up, and sending her legs overhead. He performs a squat to enter her and penetrates while keeping his arms parallel to the floor.

*AKA: The Forbidden Russian Dance.

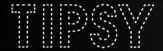

TIPSY

Her — Roll back vertebrae by vertebrae so that you are stacking your spine in a strong and supported way. Stop at your upper shoulders, you don't want to put pressure on your neck. Enjoy a strong white Russian.

Him — You might need to Putin your onion dome into her borscht before finding your deepest squat pose.

>>> THE ADVANCED DANCERS CAN RAISE ONE LEG WHILE LOWERING THEMSELVES INTO HER.

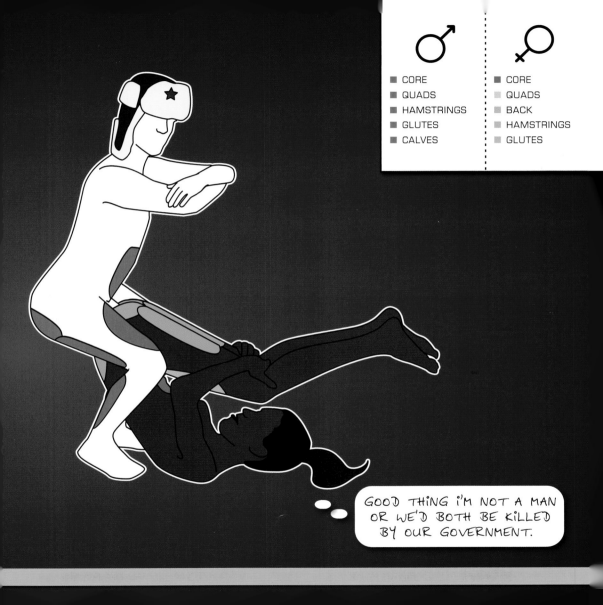

43

THE BALL BOUNCER BUILT FOR 2

He lowers his bum down into a balanced stance on the yoga ball. She straddles him and uses his penis inside her to aid in her balance. He leans back and flexes his glutes while she tries to shock his shakras.

TIPSY

Her — Pulse up and down with your inner thighs, milking him until he explodes. Or you can rock him slowly and work your tummy.

Him — You can use her hips for support. This is a hard-core core workout and we know it.

>>> HE CAN LET GO OF HER HIPS AND PLACE HIS HANDS BEHIND HIS NECK.

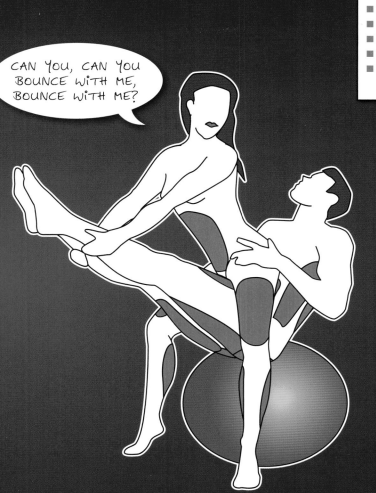

44

EAR MUFF PULL-UPS

She pulls herself up and drapes her legs on his shoulders. With his tongue working her vagina she does weight-supported pull-ups.

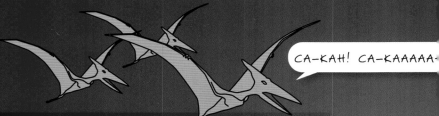

CA-KAH! CA-KAAAAA-

TIPSY

Her — If pull-ups are too difficult, even with the support of your man you can just hold yourself with flexed arms for as long as possible. He will make it worth every extra second! Be sure you moan loud enough so he can hear you. You are a thigh master.

Him — Keep your legs slightly bent for an active body. Don't ever lock your knees.

Both — Always watch your back for pterodactyl attack. But you know? It's not a bad way to go. Hold on to your butts, this is going to be a bumpy ride.

>>> **FOR ADVANCED SHE SHOULD KEEP HER LEGS UP BUT NOT LET THEM REST ON HIS SHOULDERS.**

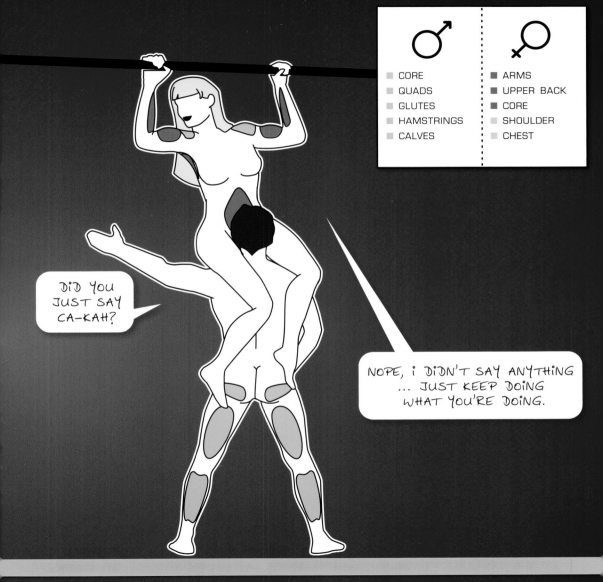

45

ROCK THE CRADLE OF LOVE

Find a comfortable chair or use the end of the bed. She should start by straddling him and then slowly move her feet onto his chest and lean back. He must make sure to hold her arms and support her in his love cradle.

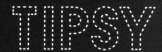

Her — Dig your feet into your man's sexy chest. Hold on tight and don't let go or you'll be dancing with yourself in a neck brace. After you rock the cradle for a while you will want to counter it with the spinxter stretch (pose 14).

Him — It's a nice day for an intense full body workout. You can stand up and thrust into your woman. If you can't stand up then do calf raises. Keep your biceps flexed and slowly bend backwards.

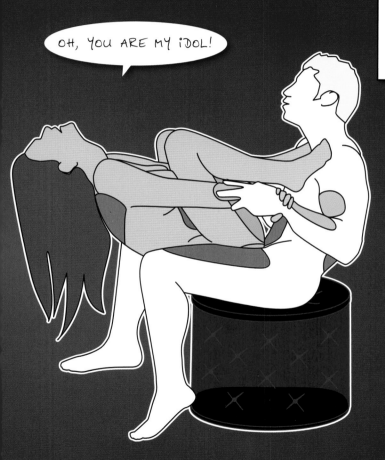

46

STIRRUPS

Ladies, when was the last time you had fun while finding yourself with feet in stirrups? And no - your last gyno visit doesn't count... Let's play doctor, the vagina kind! He goes into bridge while she leans back using his knees for support. Then he lifts her legs up so she is fully balanced on his instrument.

TIPSY

Her — The goal here is to scoop your core to engage your abs and rock back onto your tailbone with extended legs. This takes great focus, stability and strength. Use your arms to support your balance and get that extra workout.

Him — Make sure your feet and knees are parallel and hip-width apart. Scoop and tuck your tailbone beneath you for each thrust. Follow up with a child's pose to release your spine and core.

Both — Sex reduces cholesterol.

>>> **HE CAN BENCH-PRESS HER LEGS WITH RESISTANCE.**

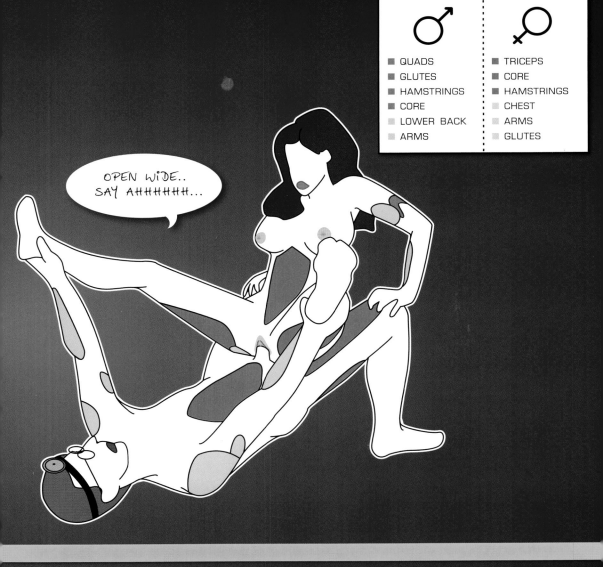

47

EAT, PRAY, HUMP

Start from Doggy Style (pose 21). He leans down, grabs her ankles and slowly raises her body. She sculpts her arms while he shreds his traps.

TIPSY

Her — Stay in this position and gently bring your legs towards your head and then back towards his thighs. Engage your core.

Him — Shrugs, hold each shrug for five seconds.

Both — Use a yoga mat to protect your knees and wrists. And an Eastern philosophy to protect your mind.

"To lose balance sometimes for love is part of living a balanced life."

Elizabeth Gilbert - "Eat, Pray, Love"

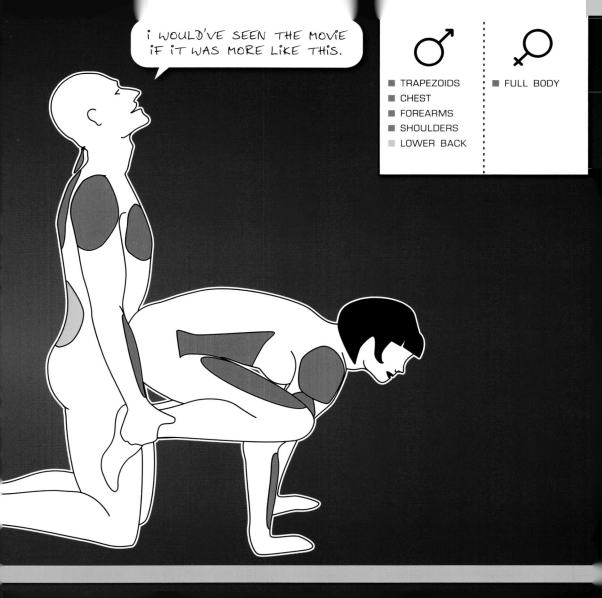

48
COITUS ARABESQUE

This prima ballerina stays after the class to spend a little time on her barre work. The teacher spots her from behind and inserts his barre into her pink tutu. She raises one leg behind her and holds it in her hand, leaving the other hand free to fondle both partners' genitals. He stands strong to keep her supported.

TIPSY

Her — Switch sides often so that you get a consistent workout on both sides of your body. Symmetry is sexy.

Him — Bend your knees to a slight squat for balance and strength training.

>>> FOR MORE ADVANCED WORKOUT SHE CAN LOWER HER HANDS TO THE FLOOR WHILE KEEPING HER LEG U

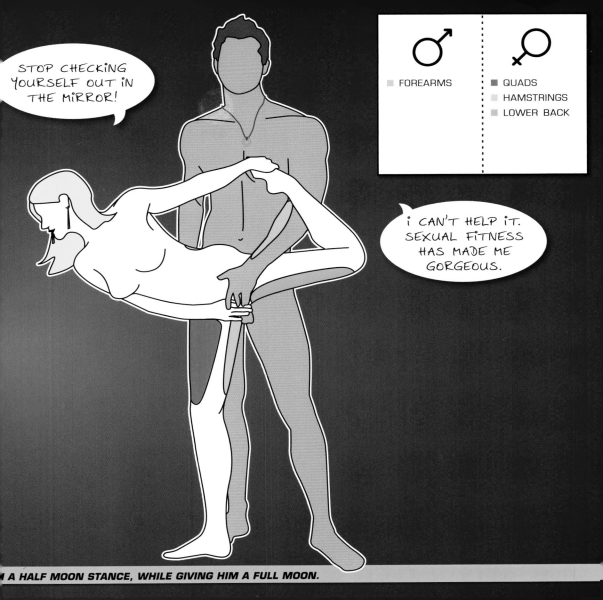

THE JAGUAR

She stalks her prey on all fours. He sits back on his legs and she extends her feet behind her. Once they find their rhythm, he raises his body up, staying inside her. She should clasp her thighs onto him to hold on and to work out. Unleash your sexy beast.

*also called: The Deep Plank.

TIPSY

Her — If you are really feeling strong, hold yourself up with one hand and cup his balls with the other. Or bring your right knee to your right elbow for five counts and then switch sides.

Him — Don't let her workout slow you down. Get in there.

FEEL FREE TO PURR AND ROAR – IT'S FUN. SHE CAN DO A PUSH-UP EVERY FIVE THRUSTS.

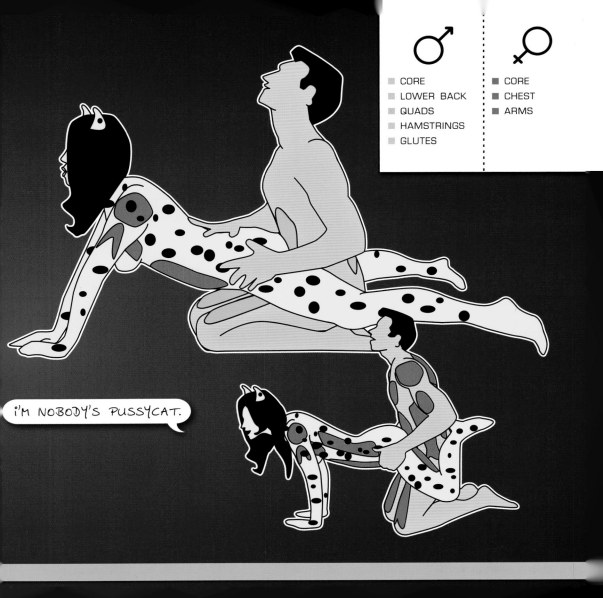

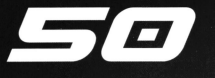

BACKSEAT DRIVER

She waits for her next fare with her hands and knees on the bed. He makes himself comfortable in her lush backseat and helps her lift her legs, wrapping them around his waist, like a seat belt. He controls the speed from the backseat. She keeps her eyes on the road until he blows his load.

TIPSY

Her — Sculpt your tummy by flexing your core muscles but be careful not to strain your back. You can also switch back and forth between elbow and push-up position to enhance your core workout. Nice interior!

Him — Plant your feet just wider than your shoulders and perform squats and calf raises in between thrusts. The lower the squat the better.

>>> HE SHOULD SLOWLY ROTATE HIS HIPS TO ADD TO HIS WORKOUT AND ADD TO HER PLEASURE AT THE SAME TIM

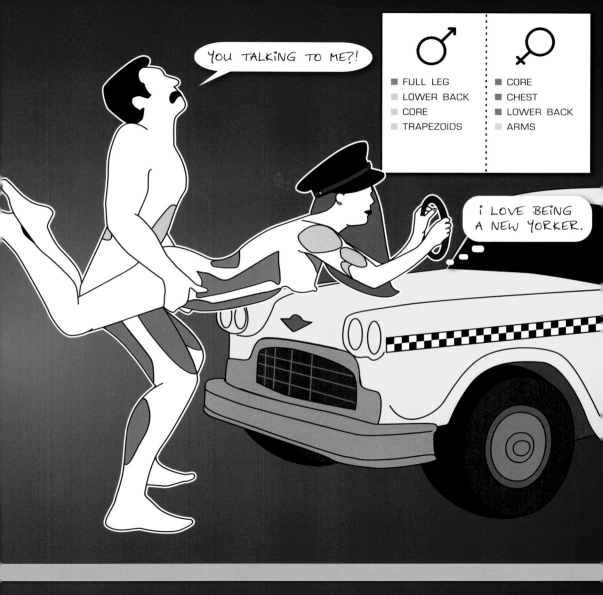

THE HOWLING WOLF

He starts on his back under her full moon. She slides his wolf man shaft inside her love den and arches her back while he pushes them up using his tricep muscles. Feel the burn and let it out in an orgasmic howl!

TIPSY

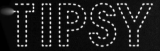

Her — Flex your abs and hold your arms parallel to the floor, think of a helicopter cuming in for a landing. You can get a great leg workout by only doing squats on his cock. Concentrate on your balance.

Him — Keep fingers pointed towards your toes. Go down deep for a nice hip flexors and full leg stretch.

THIS POSE CAN BE SO EXHAUSTING THAT YOU MAY WANT TO GO INTO HIBERNATION AFTERWARDS.

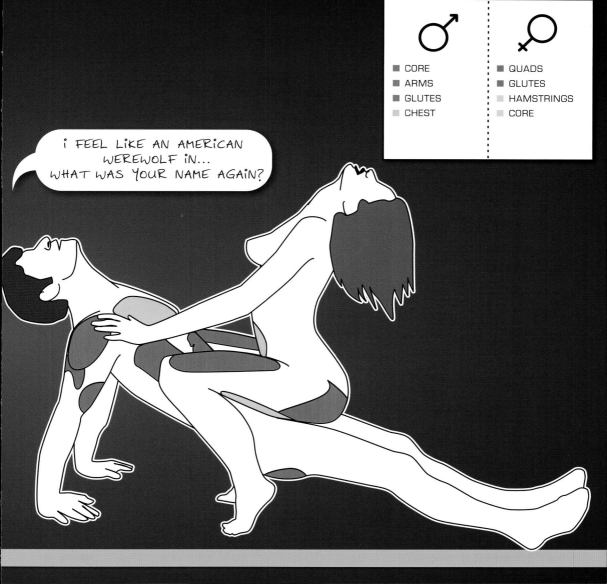

52

HOP ON COCK

MOVING HER **HIPS** FROM LEFT TO RIGHT
KEEPING HIM HARD WHILST KEEPING HER **TIGHT**
THIS SEDUCTIVE **DANCE** GETS EVEN **BETTER**
MAKING HER WHO-WHO EVEN **WETTER**
BY LIFTING A **LIMB** INTO THE AIR
UNTIL THE STRAIN YOU CANNOT BEAR
AND HE SPURTS HIS SPUNK **EVERYWHERE**
BUT YOU HAD **FUN** SO YOU DON'T CARE
GO AT IT AGAIN... IF YOU **DARE**

TIPSY

Her — You can make it easier on the man by using your legs to stay light on him. Try using your vagina to actually grab his dick and pull him up to you in rhythm.

Him — Be careful to protect the wrist joints. You can clench your fists to do reverse knuckle push-ups.

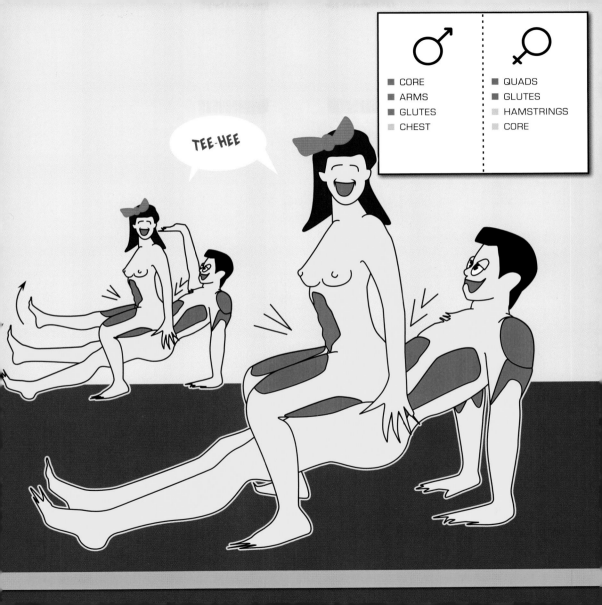

53

STARSHIP LOVE

Check out this space oddity. Han would be jealous watching the rise and fall of this starman and his princess getting layuhed. Oh, you pretty things get a great core workout in this tough pose. She lies on her back and he docks his craft in her port. Under pressure he eventually blasts off into her inner space and sends her into the cosmos.

TIPSY

Her — The more your back is off the floor or bed, the more you work out your core and lower back. This outfit will make you very popular at Comic Con.

Him — Grasp her arms and bring her body up to work your back. This will also give her a chance to decompress. Feel free to squeeze her buns.

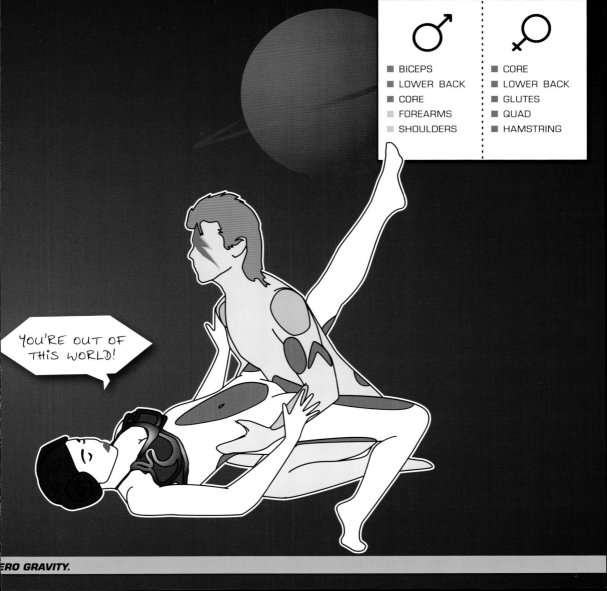

54

SEXERCISE CHAMPS OF THE WORLD!!!

In this corner, The Intimate Warrior, squaring off against the Fuck-a-maniac. Let's get readyyyyyy to hump!!! He takes her down to the mat with his signature move. He lifts her legs and wears her with pride like a championship belt.

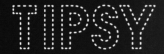

Her — Put the effort on your abs and not on your glutes. Doing dips will totally shred your arms.

Him — Support her thighs and take as much of her weight as possible. Hump hard for a great cardiovascular workout.

>>> *TO GET COMPLETELY RIPPED SHE CAN TAKE BOTH FEET OFF THE MAT AT ONCE.*

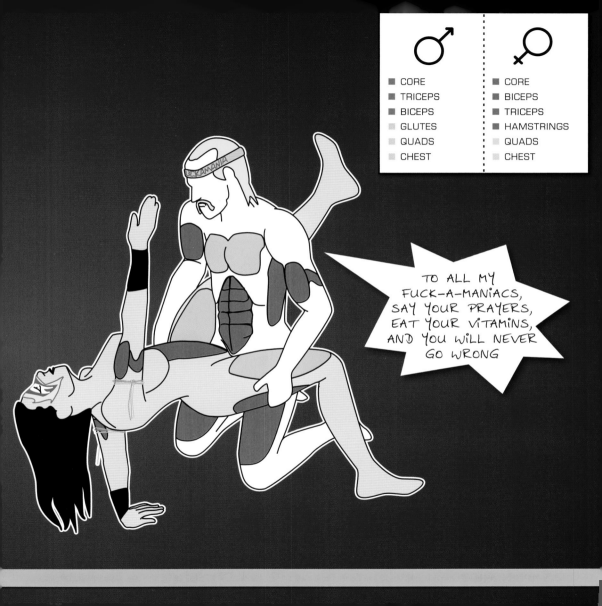

On a scale of one to ten it's like a sixty-nine

CIRQUE DU FUCK

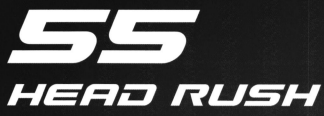

55
HEAD RUSH

To get into this pose she starts in downward dog and kicks her legs up. He holds and lifts her legs till her body is vertical. There she does shoulder presses while he supports her weight from her ankles. Blood rushes to both of their heads, her big head, his little one. Inversions are a great way to relieve the stress gravity puts on your back.

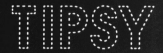

Her — Keep your back straight and your core engaged throughout the lift. Be aware of the blood flowing to your head. Come down slowly, you may get dizzy.

Him — Hold her legs firmly and be careful to help keep her aligned. Never let her twist in this pose. Suck her toes!

>>> FOR THE MOST ADVANCED HE CAN LET GO OF HER LEGS AND JUST SPOT HER OR LICK HER PUSSY IF THE

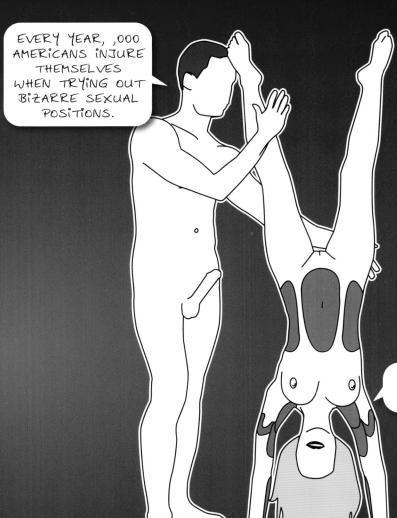

56

THE HUMAN TELESCOPE

She starts in the Head Rush (pose 55) position. He squats until his shoulders are in line with her hips. He wraps his arms around her and stands, lifting her up. She then wraps her hands around his hips to take weight off his arms and transfer more of her weight to his legs. Then they please each other orally until she tastes his Milky Way.

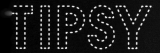

TIPSY

Her — Wait until your partner is stable before taking his junk in your mouth to avoid Bobbitation. We didn't name this pose "The Missing Sausage and the Cracked Skull" for good reason.

Him — Careful not to drop her on her head! And don't squeeze her too tight or she might bite off your rocket ship.

HE CAN DO CALF RAISES OR SPREAD HIS FEET AND DO MINI SQUATS.

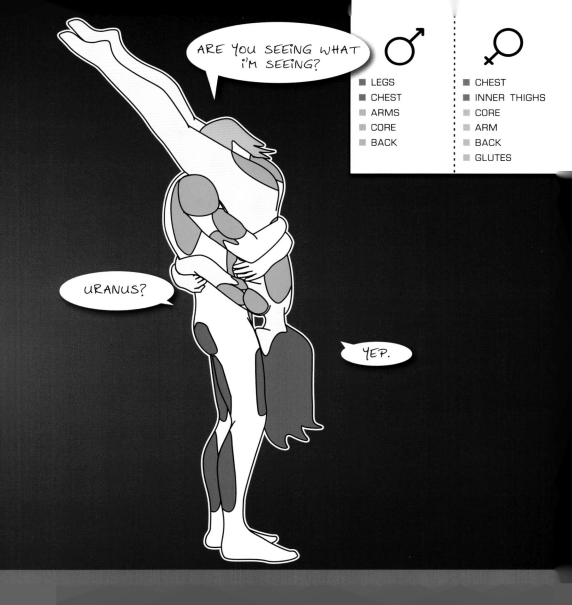

57
THE WHEEL POSE

On her back with her hands by her ears and her feet flat on the floor, knees raised, she pushes up and he slides in between her legs. Using his arms, knees and even his member, he supports the weight of his partner.

TIPSY

Her — Come down slowly by tucking your chin and slowly bending your knees until your back slowly hits the floor. Did we say slowly? The wildly advanced female can move into a full hand-stand position as he eats her out.

Him - You must act as a spotter making sure to not bang her too hard causing possible injury or death.

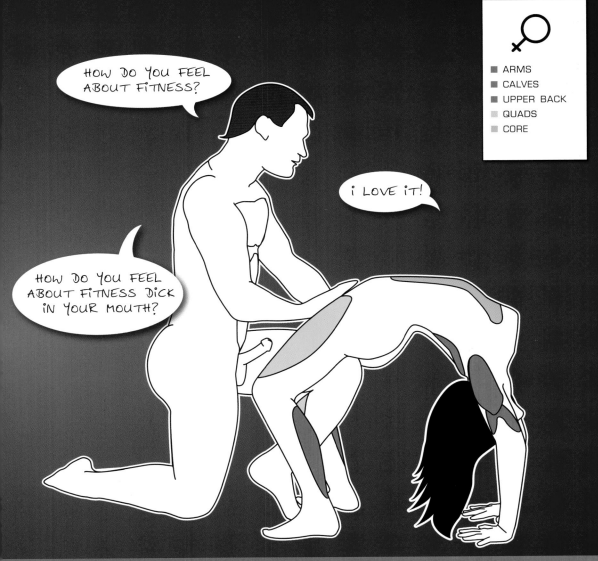

58

CROTCHING TIGER HORNY DRAGON

He does a back bridge. She crouches deeply while choking his little fire breather. Be sure to wash up after because even though man juice is good for your skin, when it dries it turns into scales.

TIPSY

Her — Do nice, smooth, slow squats. Take five seconds to get to the bottom, hold for five seconds, take five seconds to rise and hold for five seconds at the top. Repeat until he spits his flame.

Him — Men tend to not have the flexibility of women. If this is not the pose for you and you don't have wires to help you then try a low bridge with your shoulders on the floor or bed. Be careful not to break your back or strain your neck!

IF HE IS FEELING WILD, HE CAN LIFT ONE LEG PARALLEL TO THE GROUND IN SYNC WITH HER SQUATS.

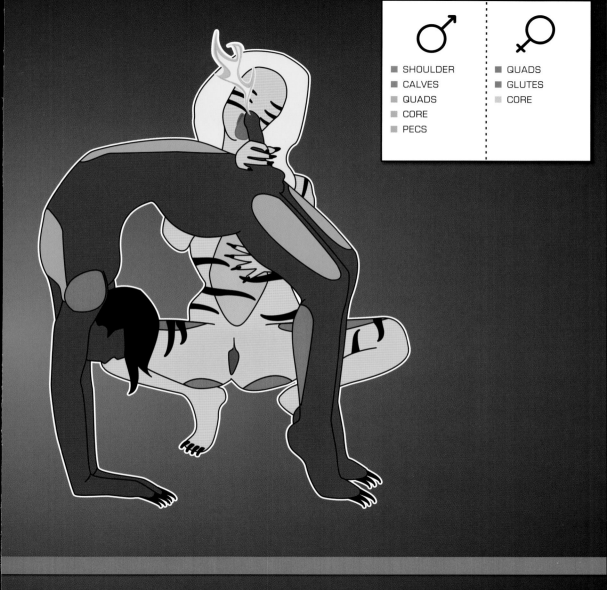

59

DOUBLE DIP*

Standing face to face he places his arms around her back. He lowers her down in a deep supported back bend. She exposes her guacamole and he dips his chip.

*also called: Bending Over Backward for Her Man.

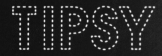

TIPSY

Her — You can use a couch, table or chair to decrease the intensity of the stretch.

Him — Keep your core engaged and isolate your glutes to pump her with your purple-headed yogurt slinger.

>>> A SUPER FREAK CAN WRAP HER LIFTED LEG AROUND HIS BACK AND PULL THEIR BODIES TOGETHER.

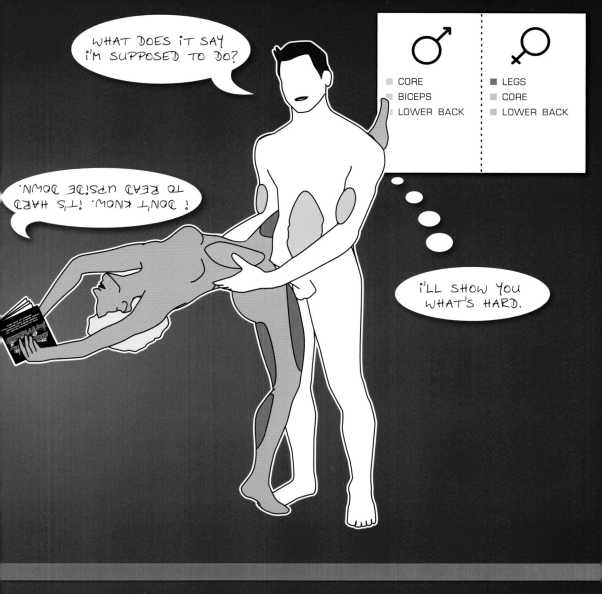

60

THE LUNGE AND PLUNGE

He slips it into her while they are both standing and facing each other. He helps her into a back bend. She lifts one leg over his shoulder. He supports her weight and plunges his hips forward in slow lunges. Boning a gymnast has its perks.

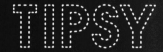

Her — You must be very conscious of your body. Breathe deeply and slowly. Do not stay in this pose for longer than you feel that you can handle it. Be the first on your block to invertedly rock that cock.

Him — Keep your knee as far forward as possible to shred your legs and abs. Hump slowly.

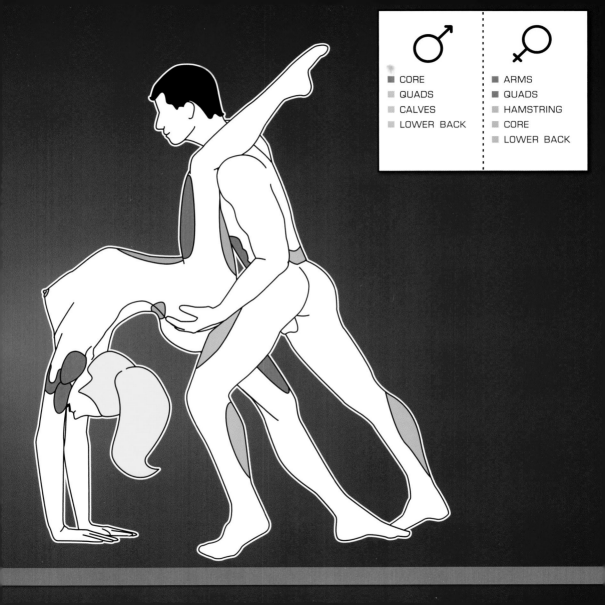

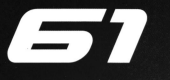

61

THE DRINKING FOUNTAIN

Using him for support, she raises into a forearm hand stand. Once she is stable she can open her legs into a front split and get slurped, sipped, licked, sucked and deep-tongue fucked.

TIPSY

Her — It's sometimes helpful to find your arm stance first against a wall. Keep your abs tight. Scissor your legs back and forth for an intense core workout. Your head, neck and spine need to stay in alignment to avoid injury.

Him — Bend your knees and activate a high lunge. Protect your knees by not letting them drift beyond your front toes and protect your back by keeping your hips squared. Get a great tongue workout. Did you know the tongue is one of the strongest muscles in the human body? Well, it is.

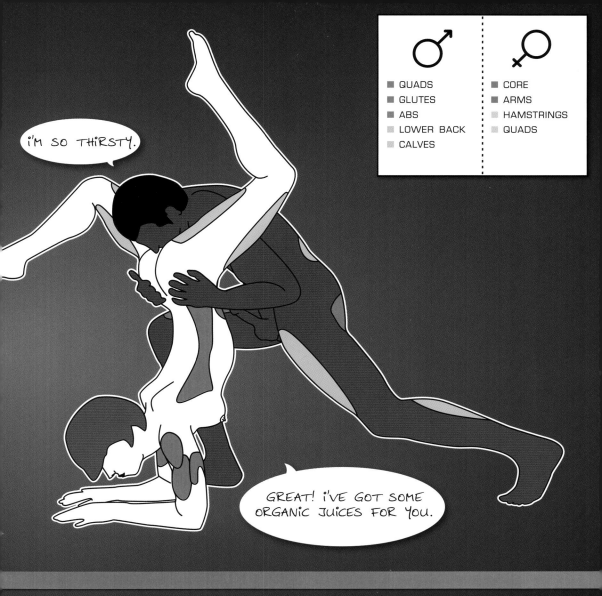

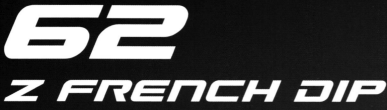

62
Z FRENCH DIP

She lays down on the bed and raises her feet in the air. Standing on the floor at the edge of the bed he inserts le penis into la vagina. She drapes her legs over his shoulders and slowly they move her arms to the floor. As they say in France: A penis is ard to find.

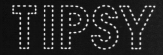

Her - Take it slow! This is an extremely hard pose, don't hurt yourself. Put something soft like a pillow under your head to make for a soft landing.

Him - You must have good balance to support her weight and not injure her.

* Literally translated - "not bad", this phrase can mean anything from "okay" to "fucking great!" It's up to you.

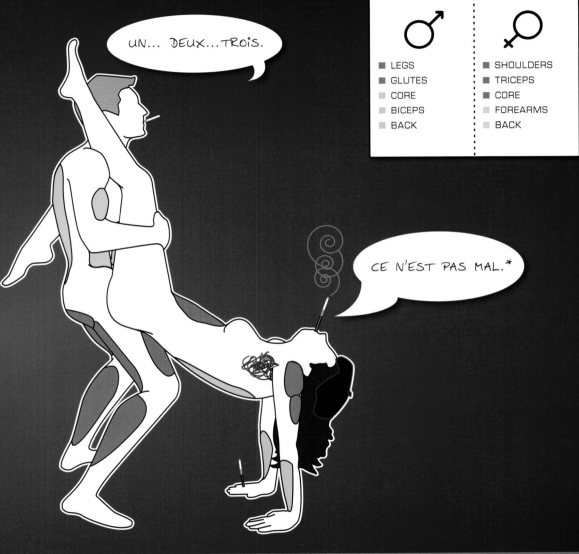

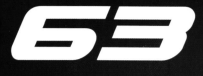

63

UPRIGHT WALL BANG

With her back against the wall, he lifts her up and lowers her down on his knob. Together they keep their neighbors awake for as long as his dong and his legs will hold out.

*also called: The Floating Scissors, The Ram, The Jerry McGuire.

TIPSY

Both — The Upright Wall Bang was made popular in the cinema of the 70's and 80's. Often followed by a clumsy stumble to the kitchen sink or dryer. In real life always choose the dryer. The faucet in the sink can leave a bruise on your glutes. If you choose to stay in the bedroom - he can step away from the wall and she can use her hips to grind out a gnarly workout. Then head back to the wall for extra support. When humping on the wall they can turn the room into a sex disco as they flick the light switch on and off with her groovy booty. Beware of wall burn!

>> IF THE WOMAN CLASPS HER LEGS TIGHTLY SHE WILL GET AN EVEN BETTER FULL BODY WORKOUT.

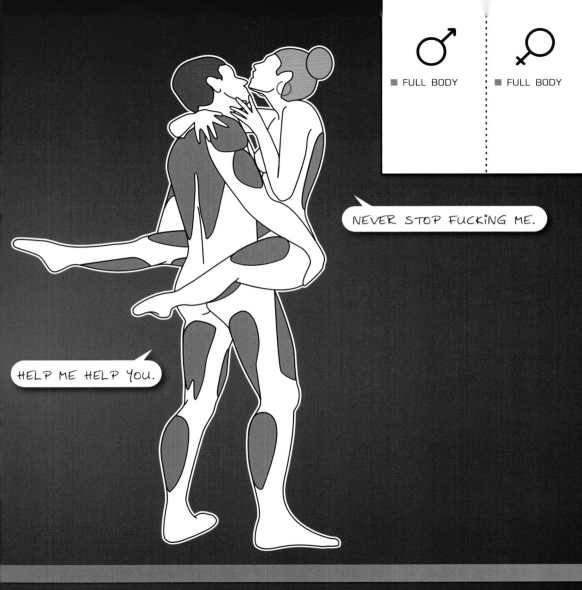

64

THE WATERFALL

From the Upright Wall Bang (pose 63) he holds her and helps her lower her hands to the ground. Deep breaths and deep penetration. You'll make a big splash at the next swingers' party if you can actually pull this one off.

TIPSY

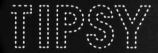

Her — Trust your partner. This is like a trust exercise. He should be there to support your weight and protect your head. Maybe have a pillow beneath you, just in case. This pose is just for special occasions.

Him — Be there to support her weight and protect her head. Instead of thrusting forward and back do calf raises and dip your noodle into the deep end of her pool. Wrap your arms around her core and lift her up for an insane full body workout.

FOR A RIDICULOUSLY HARD-CORE WORKOUT SHE CURLS HER BODY UP TO FACE HIM, THEN ROLLS BACK DOWN

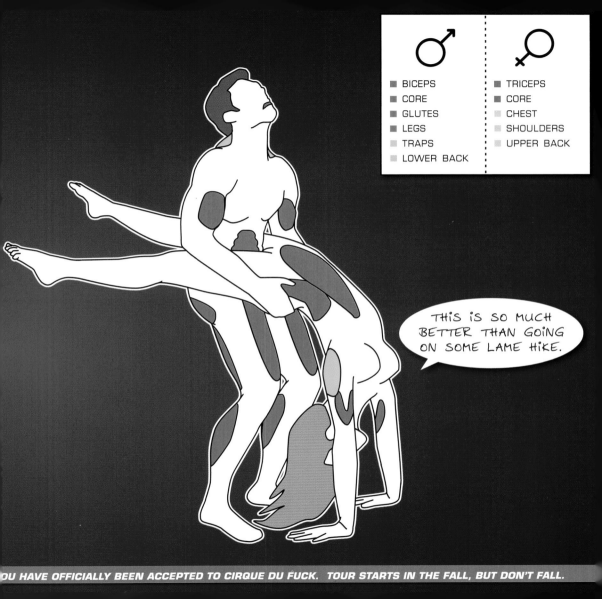

65

FLYING BUTTRESS

His feet are on the floor. She is on her hands and knees on the bed. She backs up until she is able to wrap her legs around him, like a wheelbarrow. Gently and with the utmost support she rises like a bare-breasted mermaid figurehead atop his bowsprit, surfing the supple waves of his manhood until the sea-brine splash climax.

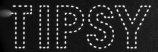

History — The Flying Buttress originated with Gothic architecture and is cum-prized of four key cum-ponents:

First, a massive erect block called the "buttress" (played by him), which is connected to the "quadrant arch" (his cock) which bridges the "gap" (her coochie-snorcher) while suspending a body between the buttress and the wall pushing outward, the "flyer" (or her).

This could end up being a religious experience! Just pray nobody gets hurt.

THIS IS A HIGHLY ADVANCED POSE, HELMETS COULD BE USED. WHO SAID HELMETS AREN'T SEXY??

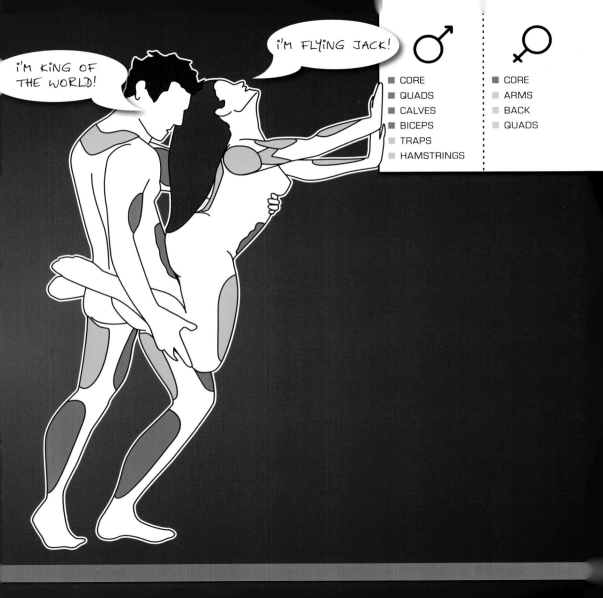

56

BOBBING FOR KNOB

Everybody loves to play dress up, so pretend everyday is Halloweenie. For those who feel like branching out - this one is for you. Dangling by her knees from a tree, pull-up bar or jungle gym (be wary of the jungle gym as coitus on a child's playground is considered a sex offense) she stretches down to take him in her mouth as he raises up on his calves, tucking his glutes and using his lower abs to thrust deep into her open throat.

TIPSY

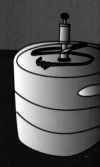

Her — Allow gravity to help you stretch out your spine. Use your abs to initiate your swing. Don't strain your neck but feel free to drain him of all fluids. Easy with the teeth.

Him — Don't go too deep! If she gags on your wanker and falls out of the tree and breaks her neck how is she supposed to suck your dick then, huh?

MAKE SURE THAT YOU ARE NOT TOO WASTED WHEN ATTEMPTING THIS POSITION.

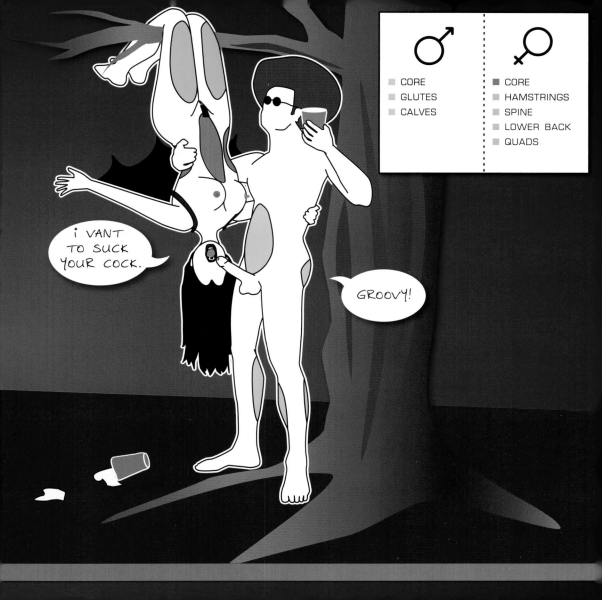

67

BANANA SPLIT WITH A CHERRY ON TOP

Congratulations! You have graduated! You are no longer sexual fitness virgins. Consider your proverbial cherries popped. Fuck it, consider yourselves Sexual Fitness Valid Dicktorians! Time for pum and circumcized. Get your just desserts. She lowers herself onto his sugar cone, working her arms and stretching her legs. He stays hard until he spurts his soft serve.

TIPSY

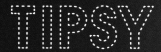

Her — You have almost made it to the end of the book. You have back-bended, deep-dipped, muff-dived, and who knows what else, but you are almost at the finish line. Just enjoy this pose and feel free to eat and cover you and your partner in loads of dark chocolate syrup.

Him — Gently lift and lower your banana by curling up your lower abs but make sure not to throw off her split balance. You have also grown through this book so you can now lift your legs nine and a half inches off the ground for an added lower ab workout.

>>> YOU ARE SO CLOSE, JUST DON'T DROP YOUR DIPLOMA BEFORE THE FINAL TEST.

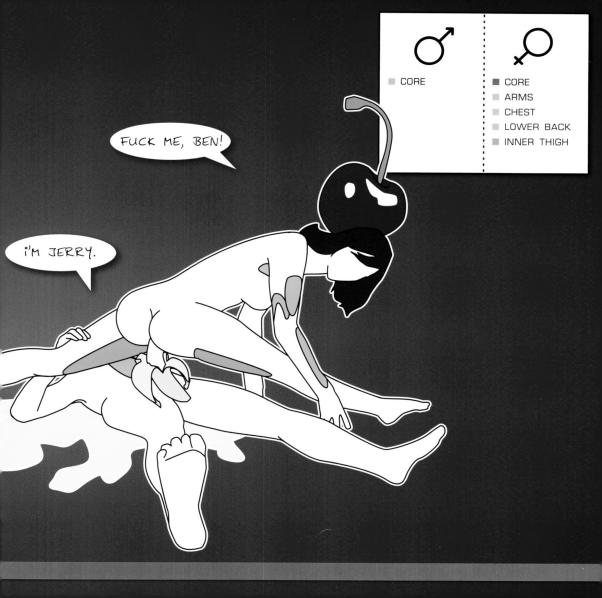

68

OUROBOROS

Ouroboros means "the snake eating its own tail" and it is a symbol that dates back to ancient Egypt. It represents renewal. Since the beginning of time man has been trying to suck his own dick. Very few will reach but those who try will get an awesome stretch in their upper back and neck.

TIPSY

Him — Surgically removing your lower ribs will help you get there. If that doesn't work then penile extension surgery could do the trick. Still, no guarantee that you will be nuts deep in your own talk hole but at least you can show off your new big shlong.

Her — Enjoy the night off.

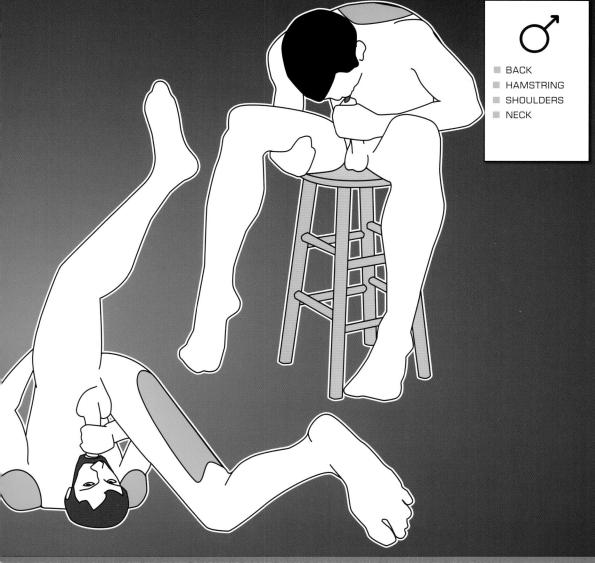

NUS. YEAH, IF YOU WANT TO TAKE SUCKING YOUR OWN COCK TO THE NEXT LEVEL GO FUCK YOURSELF.

69
GROUP SEX*

Where to begin? Invite your 50 closest Craig's List friends. The first person to arrive lies down, the last person stands up, the rest do bar dips, deep squats, circle jerks, push-ups, sit-ups, fuck-ups, suck-ups, shoulder extensions, hand-jobs, deep throat stretches, rim jobs, etc, etc, etc.

*AKA: Orgy, The 75-Headed Centipede, The Daisy Chain, Mike's Bachelor Party in Tijuana.

TIPSY

Wear a condom!
You never want to be the lazy one in a group fuck. It may be fun at the beginning, but you create habits that can last a lifetime, and before you know it you are the guy sitting on the sidelines with a camera in one hand and your dick in the other. Don't be that guy...or girl.

It's easy to not be lazy...
lift, stretch, push, and pull your way to the finish line. You will not only shred your abs but some hot members of the oppo-site sex as well.

Slow and steady wins the race in a group fuck.

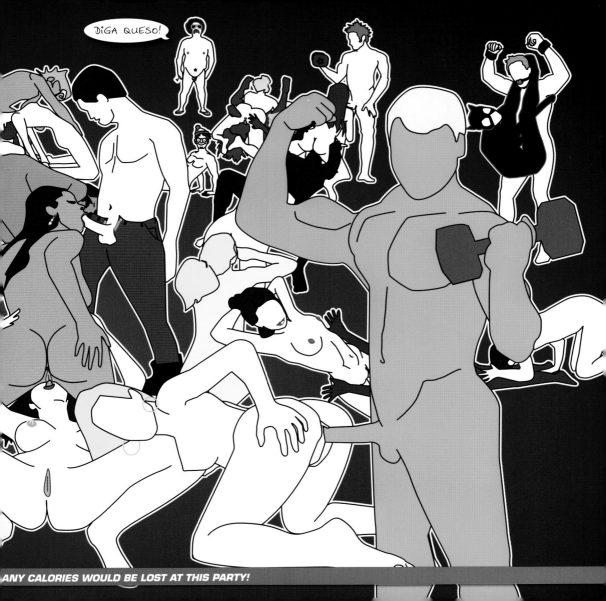

CONGRAT

LATIONS!

You have made it through the entirety of the SEXUAL FITNESS workouts. Feels good, doesn't it? You have had your ups and downs and your ins and outs and you have cum out on top. Give yourself and your partner a nice firm pat on the ass for your efforts. On the next page you will find a suggested diet, a calendar for sexual fitness goals and workouts in which different poses are matched up so that you can focus on the muscle groups you want to sculpt the most. Each series of poses will take you through a stretch and a warm-up and will lead to an intense workout of a specific muscle group. All will work your core, but you can also work a certain series one day and a different series the next so that you allow your muscles to regenerate. You are welcome to take it a step further and create your own regimen of exercises that best fits your personal desires. And most importantly, have fucking fun with it, because great sex is the best medicine.

For more go to www.sexualfitness.co.

SEXY DIET

For maximum performance you need a healthy diet that supports you sexual workout routine. If you have sex once a day, then you should hav 4 small to mid-size meals a day. If you have sex 2-4 times a day then yo should have 5-7 small to mid-size meals. If you feel that you do not hav enough time for that then you can always combine eating and sex unless you are having sex in the pool, in that case you must wait 30 min utes after you eat to avoid cramping.

It's best to have at least 35 minutes of sexual fitness daily. If you don't ge hat time in, then we recommend exercising outside of the bedroom too

FOOD FOR SEXUAL THOUGHT

PROTEINS
Fish, chicken, turkey, tofu, vegetables, vegan protein shakes.

CARBOHYDRATES
Vegetables, fruits, yams, oats,
quinoa.

OH, SO GOOD FATS
Almonds, walnuts, cashews, avocado, coconut oil, olive oil.

SEX-BOOSTING SUPPLEMENTS
ZMA, BCAAs, glutamine, fish oil,
deer antler, chlorophyll,
multi-minerals

"Your body is not a temple, it's an amusement park. Enjoy the ride."

Anthony Bourdai

Eat as much fresh organic food as possible. Avoid canned or processed foods. Tuna in moderation. Stay away from salt, sugar, bread, and dairy (trust us). Drink about a gallon of water a day. Add lemon. Pineapple juice makes your semen and vagina taste better. And remember what Shakespeare taught us about alcohol and sex - it provokes the desire but takes away the performance. Be a top performer!

SAMPLE MEAL PLAN

8:00AM
Breakfast SexFest: 2-5 egg whites with your choice of green veggies. Broccoli is recommended as it boosts men's testosterone levels and women's libido. A handful of sexy strawberries on the side for healthy sugars that keep your love potions sweet.

11:00AM
Snack: Vegan protein shake or a handful of raw almonds because their scent stimulates arousal, or an avocado, an aphrodisiac that also looks like a nut sack.

1:00PM
Lunch: Salad with lean meat or vegetable-based protein, light dressing - olive oil and lemon are a great choice. Your partner does the tossing.

4:00PM
Snack: A banana, a cucumber or a fresh peach. For a workout warm-up you can imagine that the snack is your lover's genitals. Never chew your actual partner's genitals but you can swallow.

7:00PM
Dinner: Small portion of yams or asparagus and some lean meat, fresh salmon, oysters or a vegetable-based protein with a side of salad or a grain such as quinoa.

Don't eat two hours before bed unless you have some great sexual fitness and you get hungry, in which case eat a light, healthy snack, maybe even a dark chocolate-dipped strawberry, because it is healthier to cheat on your diet than your lover. And did you know there are only 5 calories in a teaspoon of sperm?

SUGGESTIVE WAYS

UPPER BODY   3   +   11   +

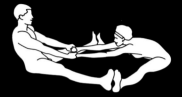 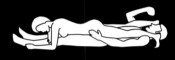

LEGS   8   +   51   +

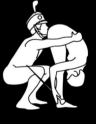 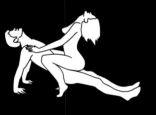

FLEXIBILITY   14   +   20   +

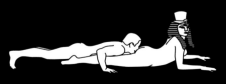 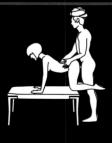

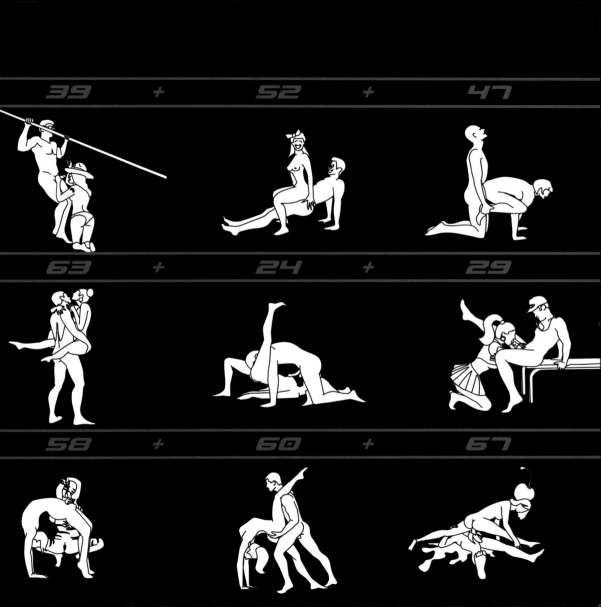

SEX CALENDAR

WEEK 1	MONDAY	TUESDAY	WEDNESDAY

WEEK 2	MONDAY	TUESDAY	WEDNESDAY

WEEK 3	MONDAY	TUESDAY	WEDNESDAY

WEEK 4	MONDAY	TUESDAY	WEDNESDAY

THURSDAY	FRIDAY	SATURDAY	SUNDAY
THURSDAY	FRIDAY	SATURDAY	SUNDAY
THURSDAY	FRIDAY	SATURDAY	SUNDAY
THURSDAY	FRIDAY	SATURDAY	SUNDAY

VAGINA

Backseat	Oasis
Beaver	Pink Cathedral
Box	Pink Taco
Borscht	Pink Tutu
Cave	Poon Tang
Cherry	Port
Coochiesnorcher	Pussy
Cookie	Sideways Smile
Crater	Silky Folds
Crotch	Snake Pit
The C word	Snatch
Flower	Sputnik
Gap	The Space Between
Genitals	Tulip
Hairy Clam	Twat
Hole	Vag
Kelp Forest	Va-Jay-Jay
Labia	Watering Hole
Love Den	Who-Who
Muff	
Netherlips	
Nook	

PENIS

Bar	Pee Pee
Bone/Boner	Peter
Carrot	Pole
Cock	Power Drill
Craft	Privates
Crotch	Rocket Ship
Dick	Sausage
Dingus	Shaft
Dong	Shlong
Flesh Sword	Skin Flute
Fire Breather	Snake
Genitals	Sugar Cone
Gun	Sumo Wrestler
Hedgehog	Third Leg
Instrument	Ting Tang
Jimi	Tonsil Tickler
Johnson	Wang
Knob	Wanker
Manhood	Whistle
Member	Woody
Mini Me	Yogurt Slinger
Onion Dome	

INTERCOURSE

Balling
Bang
Bone
Boinking
Bump Uglies
Coitus
Copulation
Fornication
Fuck
Hump
Lovemaking
Mating
Motion of the Ocean
Plunge
Pound
Pump Your Thrust
Screw
Sex
Thump
Venery

ORGASM

Avalanche
Blasts Off
Blowing Your Load
Climax
Creaming
Cum
Ejaculation
Explosion
Gee Whiz
Honorable Discharge
Jizz/Jizzum
Peek
Sploog
Spurts His Spunk
Squirts

ACKNOWLEDGMENTS

People that helped us (in nonsexual ways):

Adam Cardon
Danya Solomon
Evan Susser
Michael Homler
Mark Smylie
The Peled Brothers
Rona Sagi
Sean Burgess
Van Robichaux

THANK YOU!

Thank you for playing. Thank you to our partners, past and present, you taught us everything we know.

WHERE WE CUM FROM

Lee is D.J.'s little brother, so growing up he got lots of hand-me-down porn to help him grow his sexual understanding. D.J. and Marc were roommates in college. At school D.J. taught Marc his first words in Hebrew: "Tochlee et ha betsim shelli" (Translation: Eat my balls). Marc used that phrase on his first date with Anat and it worked. She didn't eat his balls but she thought he was funny and they all lived happily ever after. Writing a sex book together just seemed to fit the natural progression for everyone.

D.J. GUGENHEIM
FAVORITE POSE: 12

D.J. Gugenheim grew up in New York, Israel and Florida. At 16, he moved to LA by himself to pursue a girl, which needless to say didn't go well - if only he knew then what he knows now about Sexual Fitness. Despite this itinerant lifestyle, he was admitted to UCLA a year early and studied theater and business. There, he won the Gilbert Cates award for outstanding production. He worked at the Woodrow Wilson Center and on Capitol Hill. He worked for the filmmaker Joel Zwick (MY BIG FAT GREEK WEDDING) and used that experience to produce a short film with Kenan Thompson (SNL). Following that, he worked at CAA, Paramount Vantage and the Universal–based production company responsible for the BOURNE IDENTITY franchise. He runs production and development for the indie film company behind THE KIDS ARE ALRIGHT, THE GREY, KILLING THEM SOFTLY and GRACE OF MONACO. Throughout his quest to tell great stories and enjoy life and love, it became apparent to him that everyone could feel better and be happier if they had more sex and more exercise and so he decided to find the right partners to share with people a simple and fun way to engage in Sexual Fitness.

ANAT EREZ-FELLNER AND MARC FELLNER-EREZ

ANAT'S FAVORITE POSE: 53
MARC'S FAVORITE POSE: 66

Anat was born and raised in Israel. She moved to New York in 2001, where she studied package design at the Fashion Institute of Technology. She is a graphic designer and an artist.

Marc was born on the island of Guam and reached puberty in Northern California. He received his BA and his MA from UCLA's School of Theater, Film and Television. Marc is an actor, an artist and a writer.

The two met at the Brooklyn Museum on Marc's 27th birthday and got married 8 months later. They have traveled all over the world and have lived in New York and the Caribbean. They now live together in Los Angeles with their son, Brooklyn, and their pussycat, Oscar. They both appreciate that if it weren't for sex they never would have been born. Marc and Anat hope their parents are proud of their first published book. Live, love, laugh and be happy.

LEE ASHER

FAVORITE POSE: 25

Lee Asher was born in New York City and grew up in South Florida. He went to Arizona State University, where he opened up his own gym that focused on functional training. After graduating and traveling through Eastern Europe he became Tony Robbins' #1 peak performance strategist. He is now living in Los Angeles as a corporate trainer.

www.sexualfitness.co